COMPREHENSIVE HEALTH FOR THE MIDDLE GRADES

ABSTINENCE

Dale Zevin, MA

ETR Associates
Santa Cruz, California
1996

ETR Associates (Education, Training and Research) is a nonprofit organization committed to fostering the health, well-being and cultural diversity of individuals, families, schools and communities. The publishing program of ETR Associates provides books and materials that empower young people and adults with the skills to make positive health choices. We invite health professionals to learn more about our high-quality publishing, training and research programs by contacting us at P.O. Box 1830, Santa Cruz, CA 95061-1830, (800) 321-4407.

Dale Zevin, MA, is a professional writer and trainer who has developed and delivered curriculum and training manuals for diverse audiences ranging from early childhood educators to corporate managers. Her elementary through university level experience includes positions as a junior high school Spanish teacher, bilingual education instructor, district-level coordinator, and County Office of Education Administrator of Projects and Curriculum. She is also the author of ETR Associates' *Comprehensive Health for the Middle Grades: Self-Esteem*.

Comprehensive Health for the Middle Grades
  Abstinence
  Communication and Anger Management
  Consumer Health
  Drugs
  Environmental Health
  Family Relationships
  Fitness and Hygiene
  HIV and STD
  Injury Prevention
  Nutrition and Body Image
  Peer Relationships
  Puberty and Reproduction
  Self-Esteem
  Tobacco
  Violence

Printed in the United States of America

10 9 8 7 6 5 4 3 2 1

Series Editor: Kathleen Middleton

Text design: Graphic Elements

Illustrations: Ann Smiley

Title No. H565

CONTENTS

CONTENTS

CONTENTS

CONTENTS

ACKNOWLEDGMENTS

Comprehensive Health for the Middle Grades was made possible with the assistance of dedicated curriculum developers, teachers and health professionals. This program evolved from *Into Adolescence*, the middle school component of the *Contemporary Health Series*. The richness of this new program is demonstrated by the pool of talented professionals involved in both the original and the new versions.

Developers

Dale W. Evans, HSD, CHES
Health Science Dept.
California State University, Long Beach

Catherine S. Golliher, PhD
Walter Reed Middle School
North Hollywood, California

Anita Hocker, EdD
School Board of Sarasota County
Sarasota, Florida

Jory Post, MA
Happy Valley Elementary School
Santa Cruz, California

Emogene Fox, EdD, CHES
Health Education Dept.
University of Central Arkansas, Conway

Janet L. Henke
Old Court Middle School
Randallstown, Maryland

Lisa K. Hunter, PhD
Health & Education Communication Consultants
Berkeley, California

Judith K. Scheer, EdS, CHES
Contra Costa County Office of Education
Walnut Creek, California

Mary Steckiewicz Garzino, MEd
Educator and Developer of Curriculum
Chicago, Illinois

Russell G. Henke, MEd
Montgomery County Public Schools
Rockville, Maryland

Susan J. Laing, MS, CHES
Dept. of Veterans Affairs Medical Center
Birmingham, Alabama

Mae Waters, PhD, CHES
Florida Dept. of Education
Tallahassee, Florida

Susan Giarratano, EdD
Health Science Dept.
California State University, Long Beach

Jon W. Hisgen, MS
Pewaukee Public Schools
Pewaukee, Wisconsin

Carole McPherson, MA
Mission Hill Junior High School
Santa Cruz, California

Dale Zevin, MA
Educational Consultant
Santa Cruz, California

Reviewers and Consultants

Robinette J. Bacon
State Dept. of Education
Carson City, Nevada

Carol I. Bratton, MA
Walters Junior High School
Fremont, California

Donald L. Calitri, EdD, CHES
Eastern Kentucky University
Richmond, Kentucky

Jon Dore
Education Consultant
Aptos, California

Debbie Baker, MS
Wilbur D. Mills Education Cooperative
Beebe, Arkansas

Elizabeth Bumpus, MEd
Sarasota County Health Dept.
Sarasota, Florida

Peggy J. Campbell, MA
Cabell County Public Schools
Huntington, West Virginia

Claire Drew, RN, MSED
School Nurse/Health Curriculum Coordinator
Gorham, Maine

Ann Bialy
Santa Rita Union School District
Salinas, California

Nanette Burton, MA
Consultant and Family Therapist
Monte Vista, Colorado

Cal Deason, MA
Aptos Junior High School
Aptos, California

Kalvin Engleberg, MA
Oakland County Health Dept.
Pontiac, Michigan

David Birch, PhD, CHES
Dept. of Applied Health Science
Indiana University, Bloomington

Marianne Bush
Pajaro Valley Unified School District
Aptos, California

David L. Delongchamp
Northside School
Cool, California

Joyce V. Fetro, PhD, CHES
San Francisco Unified School District
San Francisco, California

Judy Boswell, RN, MS, CHES
Health Education Dept.
University of Central Arkansas, Conway

Diane Davis
D. Davis Consulting and Counseling
Bellevue, Washington

Lisa Ann DiPlacido, MS
Greater Erie Community Action Committee
Erie, Pennsylvania

Cathy Fraser
Sylvandale Middle School
San Jose, California

ACKNOWLEDGMENTS

Jaine Gilbert
King Junior High School
Berkeley, California

Gregory D. Gordon
American Indian Education and Cultural Organization
Martinez, California

Sue Gruber
Petaluma Old Adobe School
Petaluma, California

Robin McFarland Gysin
Consumer Affairs Coordinator
Santa Cruz County, California

Heidi Hataway, MS, RD
Nutritionist
University of Alabama at Birmingham

Paul G. Heller, MA, MFA
Benicia High School
Benicia, California

Anita Howard
Comprehensive Health Consultant
New Lenox, Illinois

Betty Hubbard, EdD, CHES
Health Education Dept.
University of Central Arkansas, Conway

Nina M. Jackson, MS
Fort Worth Independent School District
Fort Worth, Texas

Pam Jones, MEd
Clarksville School District
Clarksville, Arkansas

Vicki Jordan, MA
Newport Middle School
Newport, Oregon

Freya H. Kaufman, MA, CHES
Executive Consultant for School Health Programs
New York Academy of Medicine

Suzanne Kordesh, MPH, RD
Nutrition Consultant
Berkeley, California

Dan Kuhl
Wisconsin School for the Visually Handicapped
Janesville, Wisconsin

Edgar Leon, PhD
Michigan Dept. of Education
Lansing, Michigan

Linda Loushin
Junction Avenue School
Livermore, California

David M. Macrina, PhD
Dept. of Health Education and Physical Education
University of Alabama at Birmingham

Donnie McBride
Windburn Junior High
Lexington, Kentucky

Linda McDaniel, MS
Van Buren Middle School
Van Buren, Arkansas

Robert McDermott, PhD
College of Public Health
University of South Florida, Tampa

Warren McNab, PhD
Health Education Dept.
University of Nevada at Las Vegas

Louise K. Mann, MEd, MAR
Renbrook School
West Hartford, Connecticut

Eloise L. Miller, MEd
Anoka-Hennepin District #11
Anoka, Minnesota

Cheryl Mills, PHN
Soquel Elementary School District
Capitola, California

Ken Montoya
Pasadena Unified School District
Pasadena, California

Iris A. Mudd, MEd
Stokes County School District
Sandy Ridge, North Carolina

Sue Myers, MEd
Pine Strawberry School District
Pine, Arizona

Sandy Nichols, RN, MEd
State Dept. of Elementary and Secondary Education
Jefferson City, Missouri

Joanne Owens-Nauslar, EdD
Nebraska State Dept. of Education
Lincoln, Nebraska

John Pence, PhD
Newport Middle School
Newport, Oregon

Marcia Quackenbush, MS, MFCC
AIDS Health Project
University of California, San Francisco

Chuck Regin, PhD
Health Education Dept.
University of Nevada, Las Vegas

Norma Riccobuono
La Paloma High School
Brentwood, California

Fay Catlett Sady, MPH
County Office of Education
Santa Cruz, California

Paul M. Santasieri, MA
Pinelands Regional High School District
Tuckerton, New Jersey

Murry Schekman
E. A. Hall Middle School
Watsonville, California

Barbara Sheffield, MS
Whitewater Public Schools
Whitewater, Wisconsin

William Shuey
Center for Self-Esteem
Santa Cruz, California

Janet L. Sola, PhD
YWCA of the U.S.A.
New York, New York

Susan K. Telljohann, HSD
Dept. of Health Promotion and Human Performance
University of Toledo

Marcia Thompson
New Brighton Middle School
Soquel, California

Cathy Valentino
Simon and Schuster
New York, New York

Cynthia M. Walczak
New Mexico Dept. of Health—Family Planning
Santa Fe, New Mexico

Jeanne Williams
New York City Board of Education
Brooklyn, New York

Nancy Winkler, MSE
Human Growth and Development Coordinator
Oshkosh, Wisconsin

Sandra Whitney
King Estates Junior High School
Oakland, California

Glenda M. Wood
Impact Communication, Inc.
Tallahassee, Florida

Patricia Zylius
Writer
Santa Cruz, California

PROGRAM OVERVIEW

PROGRAM GOAL

Students will acquire the necessary skills and information to make healthy choices.

Comprehensive Health for the Middle Grades consists of 15 Teacher/Student Resource books, 10 of which have corresponding *Health Facts* books and sets of posters. The *Think, Choose, Act Healthy* book rounds out the basic program. Note that there are other ancillary items available, such as additional *Health Facts* books.

- **Teacher/Student Resource Books**—These 15 books address key health topics, content and issues for middle school students. All teacher/student information, instructional process, assessment tools and student activity masters for the particular topic are included in each book.

- *Health Facts* **Books**—These reference books provide clear, concise background information to support the resource books.

- ***Think, Choose, Act Healthy***—This book provides more than 130 reproducible student activities that work hand in hand with the teacher/student resource books. They will challenge students to think and make their own personal health choices.

- **Comprehensive Health Poster Series**—These 40 instructional posters inform and provoke critical student thinking. They are a high-interest way to present simple to complex health issues.

- *Spanish Resource Supplement*—The objectives, purposes, main points, vocabulary, student activity sheets and family letters from the 15 resource books are contained in this book.

PROGRAM OVERVIEW

ORGANIZATION

Comprehensive Health for the Middle Grades		
Components		
Resource Books	**Health Facts Books**	**Posters***
Abstinence	Abstinence	4 Abstinence Posters
Drugs	Drugs	4 Drugs Posters
Fitness and Hygiene	Fitness	4 Fitness and Hygiene Posters
HIV and STD	STD	4 HIV and STD Posters
Injury Prevention	Injury Prevention	4 Injury Prevention Posters
Nutrition and Body Image	Nutrition and Body Image	4 Nutrition and Body Image Posters
Puberty and Reproduction	Sexuality	4 Puberty and Reproduction Posters
Self-Esteem	Self-Esteem and Mental Health	4 Self-Esteem Posters
Tobacco	Tobacco	4 Tobacco Posters
Violence	Violence	4 Violence Posters

Additional Resources
Resource Books
Communication and Anger Management
Consumer Health
Environmental Health
Family Relationships
Peer Relationships
Health Facts Books
Disease
Environmental and Community Health
HIV

*Each content area includes: "Myth and Fact," "Dictionary of Life," "In Your Face," and "Fred and Frieda" posters.

PROGRAM OVERVIEW

SEQUENCING

Comprehensive Health for the Middle Grades is a flexible program that will allow teachers to tailor their instruction to their own students' needs and interests. For schools planning to spiral health instruction through the middle grades, the following sequence is suggested.

Please note that this is a suggested sequence. The program is designed to be flexible and meant to be arrayed in accordance with individual school needs. It may be that a different sequence is more appropriate for your school setting.

Subject Placement by Grade Level
Grade 6
Peer Relationships
Tobacco
Family Relationships
Communication and Anger Management
Environmental Health
Grade 7
Self-Esteem
Drugs
Fitness and Hygiene
Puberty and Reproduction*
Injury Prevention
Grade 8
Violence
Abstinence
Nutrition and Body Image
Consumer Health
HIV and STD

*Puberty lessons can be taught separately as early as 4th grade.

PROGRAM OVERVIEW

SUBJECT INTEGRATION

Here are suggestions for integrating health instruction into other subjects in the middle school curriculum.

Subject	Integration Suggestion	Alternate Suggestion
Language Arts	Self-Esteem Abstinence Communication and Anger Management	Violence Peer Relationships
Science	Puberty and Reproduction* Environmental Health Drugs HIV and STD Tobacco	Nutrition and Body Image Injury Prevention Fitness Consumer Health
Home Economics	Nutrition and Body Image Consumer Health	Puberty and Reproduction* Abstinence Family Relationships
Social Issues	Peer Relationships Violence Family Relationships	Drugs Tobacco Communication and Anger Management Environmental Health HIV and STD Self-Esteem
Physical Education	Fitness and Hygiene	

*Puberty lessons can be taught separately as early as 4th grade.

PROGRAM OVERVIEW

TEACHING STRATEGIES

Each resource book is designed so you can easily find the instructional content, process and skills. You can spend more time on teaching and less on planning. Special tools are provided to help you challenge your students, reach out to their families and assess student success.

A wide variety of learning opportunities is provided in each book to increase interest and meet the needs of different kinds of learners. Many are interactive, encouraging students to help each other learn. The **31** teaching strategies can be divided into 4 categories based on educational purpose. They are Informational, Creative Expression, Sharing Ideas and Opinions and Developing Critical Thinking. Descriptions of the teaching strategies are found in the appendix.

Providing Key Information

Students need information before they can move to higher-level thinking. This program uses a variety of strategies to provide the information students need to take actions for health. Strategies include:

- anonymous question box
- current events
- demonstrations
- experiments
- games and puzzles
- guest speakers
- information gathering
- interviewing
- oral presentations

Encouraging Creative Expression

Creative expression provides the opportunity to integrate language arts, fine arts and personal experience into learning. It also allows students the opportunity to demonstrate their understanding in ways that are unique to them. Creative expression encourages students to capitalize on their strengths and their interests. Strategies include:

- artistic expression
- creative writing
- dramatic presentations
- roleplays

TEACHING STRATEGIES

Sharing Ideas, Feelings and Opinions

In the sensitive area of health education, providing a safe atmosphere in which to discuss a variety of opinions and feelings is essential. Discussion provides the opportunity to clarify misinformation and correct misconceptions. Strategies include:

- brainstorming
- class discussion
- clustering
- continuum voting
- dyad discussion
- family discussion
- forced field analysis
- journal writing
- panel discussion
- self-assessment
- small groups
- surveys and inventories

Developing Critical Thinking

Critical thinking skills are crucial if students are to adopt healthy behaviors. Healthy choices necessitate the ability to become independent thinkers, analyze problems and devise solutions in real-life situations. Strategies include:

- case studies
- cooperative learning groups
- debates
- factual writing
- media analysis
- personal contracts
- research

PROGRAM OVERVIEW

SKILLS INFUSION

Studies of high-risk children and adolescents show that certain characteristics are common to children who succeed in adverse situations. These children are called resilient. Evaluation of educational programs designed to build resiliency has shown that several elements are important for success. The most important is the inclusion of activities designed to build personal and social skills.

Throughout each resource book, students practice skills along with the content addressed in the activities. Activities that naturally infuse personal and social skills are identified.

- **Communication**—Students with effective communication skills are able to express thoughts and feelings, actively listen to others, and give clear verbal and nonverbal messages related to health or any other aspect of their lives.

- **Decision Making**—Students with effective decision-making skills are able to identify decision points, gather information, and analyze and evaluate alternatives before they take action. This skill is important to promote positive health choices.

- **Assertiveness**—Students with effective assertiveness skills are able to resist pressure and influence from peers, advertising or others that may be in conflict with healthy behavior. This skill involves the ability to negotiate in stressful situations and refuse unwanted influences.

- **Stress Management**—Students with effective stress-management skills are able to cope with stress as a normal part of life. They are able to identify situations and conditions that produce stress and adopt healthy coping behaviors.

- **Goal Setting**—Students with effective goal-setting skills are able to clarify goals based on their needs and interests. They are able to set realistic goals, identify the sub-steps to goals, take action and evaluate their progress. They are able to learn from mistakes and change goals as needed.

Program Overview

Working with Families and Communities

A few general principles can help you be most effective in teaching about health:

- Establish a rapport with your students, their families and your community.
- Prepare yourself so that you are comfortable with the content and instructional process required to teach about abstinence successfully.
- Be aware of state laws and guidelines established by your school district that relate to health.
- Invite parents and other family members to attend a preview of the materials.

Some lessons include letters about the units and activities to be completed at home. Family involvement improves student learning. Encourage family members and other volunteers to help you in the classroom as you teach these activities.

It is always important to be sensitive to the diverse family situations of your students. Be alert to family situations that may make completion of an assignment difficult for a student and make alternate arrangements as necessary.

THE ABSTINENCE RESOURCE BOOK

WHY TEACH ABOUT ABSTINENCE?

Support for sexual abstinence (voluntarily refraining from sexual intercourse) as a logical, positive choice for young people is widespread. From the state level to the federal level, government mandates have encouraged education that emphasizes that abstinence from sexual intercourse is the only protection that is 100% effective against unwanted teenage pregnancy, sexually transmitted disease, and the sexual transmission of HIV. Abstinence is free, requires no prescription or exam, is always available, is accepted religiously and morally, is reversible and has no side effects.

Adolescents and Abstinence

Young people have an urgent need for the skills and information necessary to help them make wise choices about their sexual behaviors. In the United States, more than 1 million teen pregnancies occur each year—80% of them are unplanned. Every year, 1 in 8 teens contracts a sexually transmitted disease. HIV, the virus that causes AIDS, is a danger to Americans of all ages and sexual orientations.

Students at the middle school level need time to grow up without the emotional upheavals and health risks of early sexual involvement. At this age, positive and rewarding friendships are essential; sexual relationships are not. Abstinence is the wisest and healthiest choice for students.

Students can and should make a commitment to abstinence. You can support your students by teaching them skills to help them maintain their commitment.

To promote positive health behavior, these units provide practice with a variety of communication skills—including assertiveness skills and refusal techniques—that can be used to abstain from sex. The activities provide middle school students with knowledge and skills that will help them abstain from sexual behavior, respect others' decisions to abstain from sex, and establish positive social relationships.

Background Information on Abstinence

Instant Expert sections throughout this book give you all the information you need to teach each unit.

Expressing Affection (p. 12)
Facts About Abstinence (p. 24)
Assertiveness Skills (p. 48)
Learning to Say No (p. 61)
Personal Support Systems (p. 71)

THE ABSTINENCE RESOURCE BOOK

OBJECTIVES

Students Will Be Able to:

Unit 1: Affectionately Yours
- Describe a range of behaviors that demonstrate affection.

Unit 2: Crystal Ball
- Analyze consequences of sexual intercourse for adolescents.

Unit 3: Staying Safe
- Identify uncomfortable situations and settings that may be conducive to sexual behavior.

Unit 4: Assertive Me!
- Demonstrate effective assertive communication skills.

Unit 5: Pressure Lines
- Demonstrate refusal techniques to help them resist pressures to engage in sexual activity.

Unit 6: We're There for You
- Identify personal support systems to help them abstain from sex.

ANATOMY OF A UNIT

PREPARING TO TEACH

Objective identifies what students are expected to be able to do after instruction.

Getting Started lists preparation needed, including which masters to use.

Purpose states the rationale for the unit. **Main Points** are the key issues addressed. **Review** identifies the readings to increase your expertise in the content.

Vocabulary provides definitions of words used in the unit.

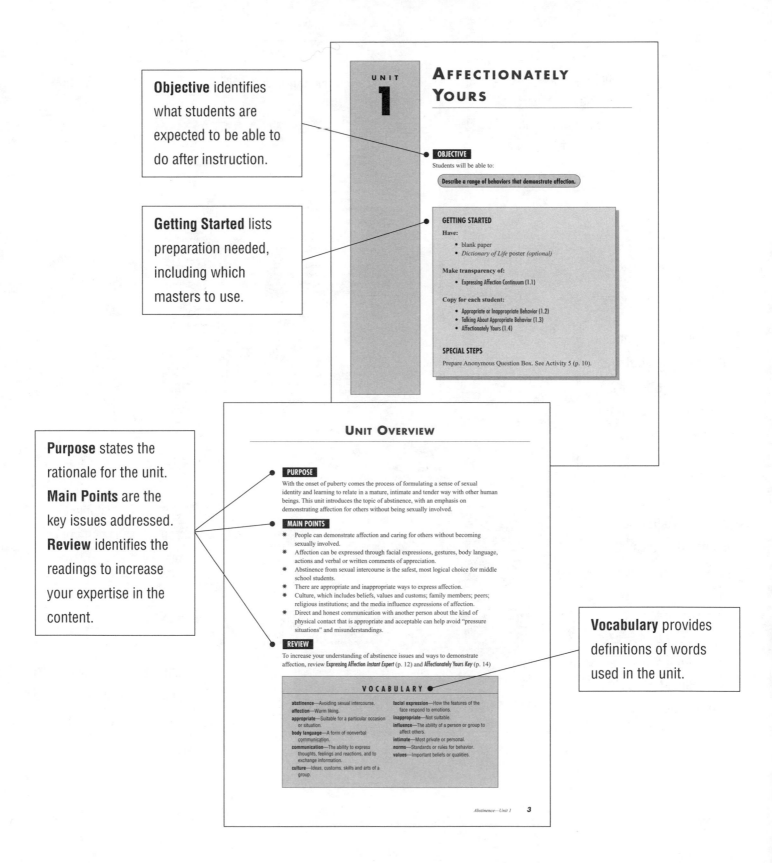

UNIT
1

AFFECTIONATELY YOURS

OBJECTIVE

Students will be able to:

Describe a range of behaviors that demonstrate affection.

GETTING STARTED

Have:
- blank paper
- *Dictionary of Life* poster *(optional)*

Make transparency of:
- Expressing Affection Continuum (1.1)

Copy for each student:
- Appropriate or Inappropriate Behavior (1.2)
- Talking About Appropriate Behavior (1.3)
- Affectionately Yours (1.4)

SPECIAL STEPS

Prepare Anonymous Question Box. See Activity 5 (p. 10).

UNIT OVERVIEW

PURPOSE

With the onset of puberty comes the process of formulating a sense of sexual identity and learning to relate in a mature, intimate and tender way with other human beings. This unit introduces the topic of abstinence, with an emphasis on demonstrating affection for others without being sexually involved.

MAIN POINTS

* People can demonstrate affection and caring for others without becoming sexually involved.
* Affection can be expressed through facial expressions, gestures, body language, actions and verbal or written comments of appreciation.
* Abstinence from sexual intercourse is the safest, most logical choice for middle school students.
* There are appropriate and inappropriate ways to express affection.
* Culture, which includes beliefs, values and customs; family members; peers; religious institutions; and the media influence expressions of affection.
* Direct and honest communication with another person about the kind of physical contact that is appropriate and acceptable can help avoid "pressure situations" and misunderstandings.

REVIEW

To increase your understanding of abstinence issues and ways to demonstrate affection, review Expressing Affection *Instant Expert* (p. 12) and Affectionately Yours *Key* (p. 14)

VOCABULARY

abstinence—Avoiding sexual intercourse.
affection—Warm liking.
appropriate—Suitable for a particular occasion or situation.
body language—A form of nonverbal communication.
communication—The ability to express thoughts, feelings and reactions, and to exchange information.
culture—Ideas, customs, skills and arts of a group.

facial expression—How the features of the face respond to emotions.
inappropriate—Not suitable.
influence—The ability of a person or group to affect others.
intimate—Most private or personal.
norms—Standards or rules for behavior.
values—Important beliefs or qualities.

Abstinence—Unit 1 **3**

ANATOMY OF A UNIT

TEACHING THE ACTIVITIES

Instant Expert pages provide concise background information for you. They follow each unit.

Process Cue identifies the teaching strategy used for the activity. Descriptions are in the Teaching Strategies appendix.

Building Skills icons identify activities that provide skill-specific practice.

Sharpen the Skill suggests ideas for more skills practice.

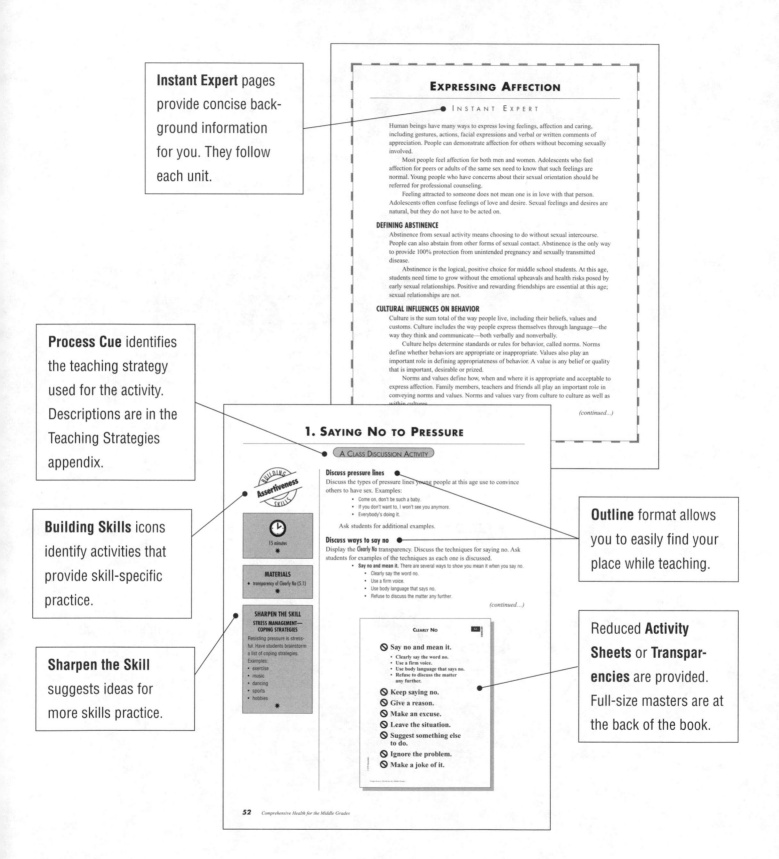

EXPRESSING AFFECTION

INSTANT EXPERT

Human beings have many ways to express loving feelings, affection and caring, including gestures, actions, facial expressions and verbal or written comments of appreciation. People can demonstrate affection for others without becoming sexually involved.

Most people feel affection for both men and women. Adolescents who feel affection for peers or adults of the same sex need to know that such feelings are normal. Young people who have concerns about their sexual orientation should be referred for professional counseling.

Feeling attracted to someone does not mean one is in love with that person. Adolescents often confuse feelings of love and desire. Sexual feelings and desires are natural, but they do not have to be acted on.

DEFINING ABSTINENCE

Abstinence from sexual activity means choosing to do without sexual intercourse. People can also abstain from other forms of sexual contact. Abstinence is the only way to provide 100% protection from unintended pregnancy and sexually transmitted disease.

Abstinence is the logical, positive choice for middle school students. At this age, students need time to grow without the emotional upheavals and health risks posed by early sexual relationships. Positive and rewarding friendships are essential at this age; sexual relationships are not.

CULTURAL INFLUENCES ON BEHAVIOR

Culture is the sum total of the way people live, including their beliefs, values and customs. Culture includes the way people express themselves through language—the way they think and communicate—both verbally and nonverbally.

Culture helps determine standards or rules for behavior, called norms. Norms define whether behaviors are appropriate or inappropriate. Values also play an important role in defining appropriateness of behavior. A value is any belief or quality that is important, desirable or prized.

Norms and values define how, when and where it is appropriate and acceptable to express affection. Family members, teachers and friends all play an important role in conveying norms and values. Norms and values vary from culture to culture as well as within cultures.

(continued...)

1. SAYING NO TO PRESSURE

A CLASS DISCUSSION ACTIVITY

Assertiveness — BUILDING SKILLS

🕐 15 minutes

MATERIALS
♦ transparency of Clearly No (5.1)

SHARPEN THE SKILL
STRESS MANAGEMENT— COPING STRATEGIES
Resisting pressure is stressful. Have students brainstorm a list of coping strategies. Examples:
• exercise
• music
• dancing
• sports
• hobbies

Discuss pressure lines
Discuss the types of pressure lines young people at this age use to convince others to have sex. Examples:
• Come on, don't be such a baby.
• If you don't want to, I won't see you anymore.
• Everybody's doing it.

Ask students for additional examples.

Discuss ways to say no
Display the Clearly No transparency. Discuss the techniques for saying no. Ask students for examples of the techniques as each one is discussed.
• **Say no and mean it.** There are several ways to show you mean it when you say no.
  • Clearly say the word no.
  • Use a firm voice.
  • Use body language that says no.
  • Refuse to discuss the matter any further.

(continued...)

CLEARLY NO

🚫 **Say no and mean it.**
  • Clearly say the word no.
  • Use a firm voice.
  • Use body language that says no.
  • Refuse to discuss the matter any further.
🚫 **Keep saying no.**
🚫 **Give a reason.**
🚫 **Make an excuse.**
🚫 **Leave the situation.**
🚫 **Suggest something else to do.**
🚫 **Ignore the problem.**
🚫 **Make a joke of it.**

52 Comprehensive Health for the Middle Grades

Outline format allows you to easily find your place while teaching.

Reduced **Activity Sheets** or **Transparencies** are provided. Full-size masters are at the back of the book.

ANATOMY OF A UNIT

SPECIAL FEATURES

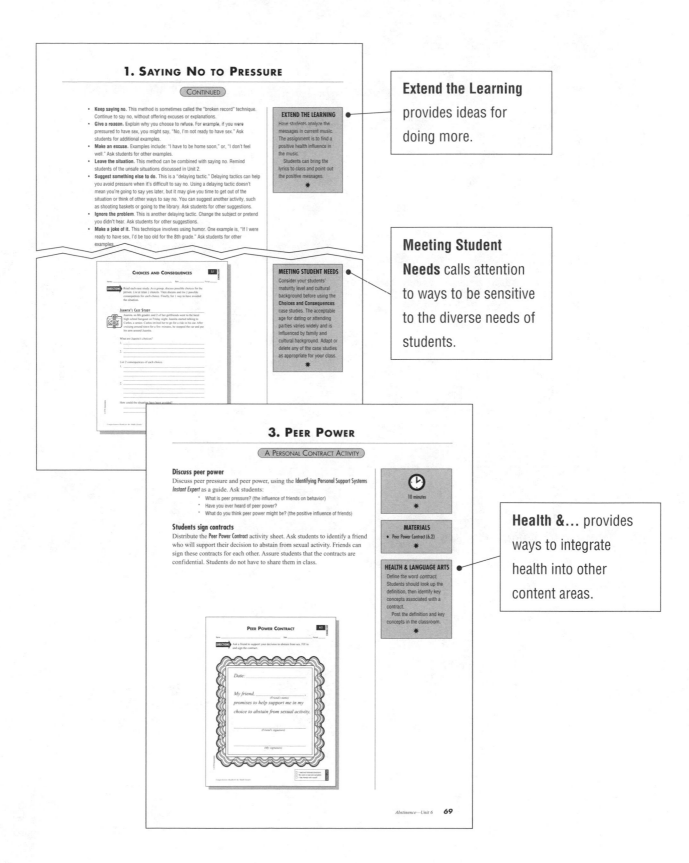

Extend the Learning provides ideas for doing more.

Meeting Student Needs calls attention to ways to be sensitive to the diverse needs of students.

Health &... provides ways to integrate health into other content areas.

ANATOMY OF A UNIT

FAMILY INVOLVEMENT

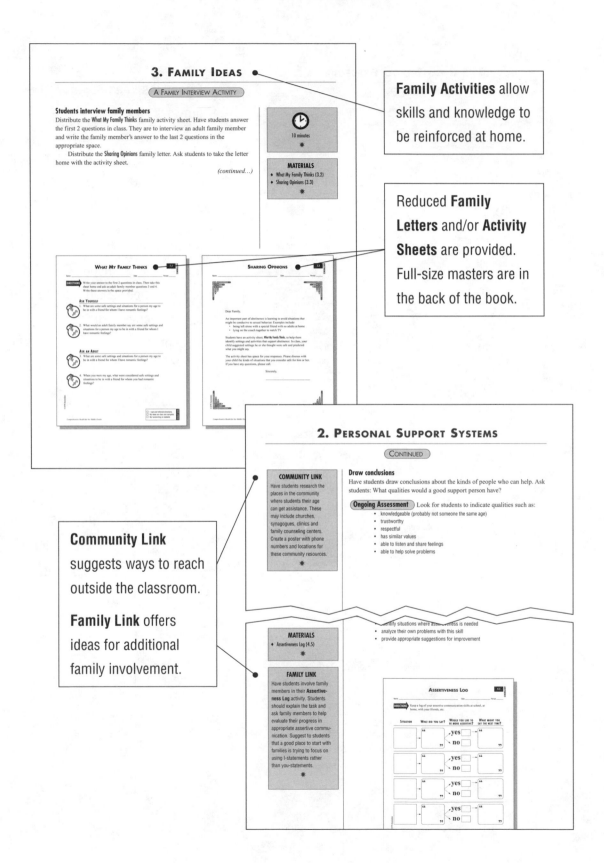

Family Activities allow skills and knowledge to be reinforced at home.

Reduced **Family Letters** and/or **Activity Sheets** are provided. Full-size masters are in the back of the book.

Community Link suggests ways to reach outside the classroom.

Family Link offers ideas for additional family involvement.

ANATOMY OF A UNIT

EVALUATION FEATURES

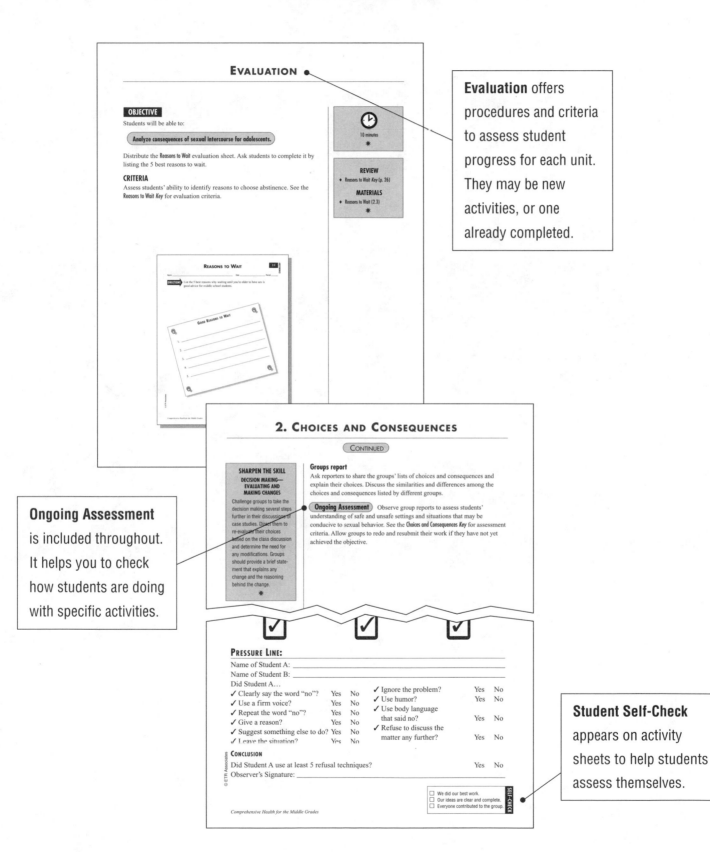

EVALUATION

Evaluation offers procedures and criteria to assess student progress for each unit. They may be new activities, or one already completed.

OBJECTIVE

Students will be able to:

Analyze consequences of sexual intercourse for adolescents.

Distribute the **Reasons to Wait** evaluation sheet. Ask students to complete it by listing the 5 best reasons to wait.

CRITERIA

Assess students' ability to identify reasons to choose abstinence. See the **Reasons to Wait** *Key* for evaluation criteria.

10 minutes

REVIEW
♦ Reasons to Wait *Key* (p. 26)

MATERIALS
♦ Reasons to Wait (2.3)

REASONS TO WAIT

DIRECTIONS List the 5 best reasons why waiting until you're older to have sex is good advice for middle school students.

GOOD REASONS TO WAIT

1.
2.
3.
4.
5.

2. CHOICES AND CONSEQUENCES

CONTINUED

SHARPEN THE SKILL

DECISION MAKING—EVALUATING AND MAKING CHANGES

Challenge groups to take the decision making several steps further in their discussions of case studies. Direct them to re-evaluate their choices based on the class discussion and determine the need for any modifications. Groups should provide a brief statement that explains any change and the reasoning behind the change.

Groups report

Ask reporters to share the groups' lists of choices and consequences and explain their choices. Discuss the similarities and differences among the choices and consequences listed by different groups.

Ongoing Assessment Observe group reports to assess students' understanding of safe and unsafe settings and situations that may be conducive to sexual behavior. See the **Choices and Consequences** *Key* for assessment criteria. Allow groups to redo and resubmit their work if they have not yet achieved the objective.

Ongoing Assessment is included throughout. It helps you to check how students are doing with specific activities.

PRESSURE LINE:

Name of Student A: _____
Name of Student B: _____
Did Student A...

✓ Clearly say the word "no"?	Yes No	✓ Ignore the problem?	Yes No
✓ Use a firm voice?	Yes No	✓ Use humor?	Yes No
✓ Repeat the word "no"?	Yes No	✓ Use body language that said no?	Yes No
✓ Give a reason?	Yes No		
✓ Suggest something else to do?	Yes No	✓ Refuse to discuss the matter any further?	Yes No
✓ Leave the situation?	Yes No		

CONCLUSION

Did Student A use at least 5 refusal techniques? Yes No
Observer's Signature: _____

☐ We did our best work.
☐ Our ideas are clear and complete.
☐ Everyone contributed to the group.

SELF-CHECK

Comprehensive Health for the Middle Grades

© ETR Associates

Student Self-Check appears on activity sheets to help students assess themselves.

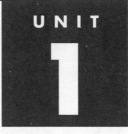

UNIT
1

AFFECTIONATELY YOURS

TIME

2 periods

ACTIVITIES

1. How Do You Show You Care?

2. Assessing Affectionate Behaviors

3. What Do Our Families Think?

4. Expressing Your Affection

5. Any Questions?

AFFECTIONATELY YOURS

OBJECTIVE

Students will be able to:

> Describe a range of behaviors that demonstrate affection.

GETTING STARTED

Have:

- blank paper
- *Dictionary of Life* poster *(optional)*

Make transparency of:

- Expressing Affection Continuum (1.1)

Copy for each student:

- Appropriate or Inappropriate Behavior (1.2)
- Talking About Appropriate Behavior (1.3)
- Affectionately Yours (1.4)

SPECIAL STEPS

Prepare Anonymous Question Box. See Activity 5 (p. 10).

UNIT OVERVIEW

PURPOSE

With the onset of puberty comes the process of formulating a sense of sexual identity and learning to relate in a mature, intimate and tender way with other human beings. This unit introduces the topic of abstinence, with an emphasis on demonstrating affection for others without being sexually involved.

MAIN POINTS

* People can demonstrate affection and caring for others without becoming sexually involved.
* Affection can be expressed through facial expressions, gestures, body language, actions and verbal or written comments of appreciation.
* Abstinence from sexual intercourse is the safest, most logical choice for middle school students.
* There are appropriate and inappropriate ways to express affection.
* Culture, which includes beliefs, values and customs; family members; peers; religious institutions; and the media influence expressions of affection.
* Direct and honest communication with another person about the kind of physical contact that is appropriate and acceptable can help avoid "pressure situations" and misunderstandings.

REVIEW

To increase your understanding of abstinence issues and ways to demonstrate affection, review **Expressing Affection** *Instant Expert* (p. 12) and **Affectionately Yours** *Key* (p. 14)

VOCABULARY

abstinence—Avoiding sexual intercourse.

affection—Warm liking.

appropriate—Suitable for a particular occasion or situation.

body language—A form of nonverbal communication.

communication—The ability to express thoughts, feelings and reactions, and to exchange information.

culture—Ideas, customs, skills and arts of a group.

facial expression—How the features of the face respond to emotions.

inappropriate—Not suitable.

influence—The ability of a person or group to affect others.

intimate—Most private or personal.

norms—Standards or rules for behavior.

values—Important beliefs or qualities.

1. How Do You Show You Care?

A BRAINSTORMING AND CLASS DISCUSSION ACTIVITY

20 minutes

MATERIALS

- transparency of Expressing Affection Continuum (1.1)
- *Optional: Dictionary of Life poster*

MEETING STUDENT NEEDS

Set up or review class groundrules before the brainstorming session. Remind students that all opinions are valid. Students should not comment about or judge other students' ideas.

Brainstorm affectionate behaviors

Ask students to think about ways they and their family members and friends demonstrate affection for each other, such as hugging. Ask students:

- What was the most recent display of affection you gave or received?
- When was it?
- Who was it with?
- What was the reason for it?

Conduct a brainstorming session to identify ways people show their affection for each other. List students' responses on the board. Responses may include:

- smiling
- hugging
- putting an arm around a shoulder or waist
- holding hands
- kissing
- spending time together
- doing things for each other

- sharing experiences
- writing cards and letters
- telephoning
- giving gifts
- confiding in each other
- being honest with each other
- sexual contact

(continued...)

EXPRESSING AFFECTION CONTINUUM   1.1   ABSTINENCE

Physical Expressions of Affection

most intimate

least intimate

© ETR Associates

Comprehensive Health for the Middle Grades

1. How Do You Show You Care?

Ask students: Which of these ways would be appropriate ways to demonstrate affection for special friends?

Students analyze physical expressions of affection

Display the Expressing Affection Continuum transparency. Ask students to identify the physical expressions of affection in the list they brainstormed in Activity 1 (smiling, kissing, hugging, putting arms around each other, holding hands). Ask students:

- Where would each of these actions go on the continuum?
- Which action is least intimate?
- Which action is most intimate?

Use students' responses to fill in the continuum on the transparency. See the Expressing Affection *Instant Expert* for an example.

Define *abstinence*

Write the word ABSTINENCE on the board. Ask students what this word means (doing without something by one's own choice). The word can refer to doing without food, drink or other pleasures, but it is frequently used to describe the decision to refrain from sexual intercourse.

Explain that students will be learning about abstinence. These units will help students understand why abstinence from sexual intercourse is the safest, most logical choice for people their age.

Ongoing Assessment   Look for student understanding of the meaning of the word *affection,* and that the expression of affection varies greatly depending on things such as:

- the relationship (parent/child, friend/friend, etc.)
- how well people in the relationship know each other
- the culture, norms and values people bring to the relationship

---

EXTEND THE LEARNING

Display the *Dictionary of Life* poster for students to use as a reference throughout this program.

✳

---

2. ASSESSING AFFECTIONATE BEHAVIORS

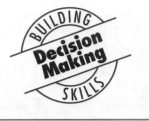

25 minutes

✸

MATERIALS

◆ Appropriate or Inappropriate Behavior (1.2)

✸

Discuss influences on behavior

Discuss the variety of influences on behavior, including cultural influences, using the **Expressing Affection** *Instant Expert* as a guide. Ask students for examples of some specific people and things that influence their behavior. Responses may include:

- parents
- siblings
- peers
- religious organizations
- TV

- movies
- videos
- music
- books
- magazines

(continued...)

APPROPRIATE OR INAPPROPRIATE BEHAVIOR **1.2** ABSTINENCE

Name _____   Date _____   Period _____

DIRECTIONS Read each item. Circle the **A** if the behavior is an appropriate way to express affection toward a special friend. Circle the **I** if it is inappropriate.

1. Ask someone to dance at the school dance.   **A** **I**

2. Hold hands at a party.   **A** **I**

3. Kiss in the school hallway.   **A** **I**

4. Knock a person's books on the floor.   **A** **I**

5. Write a message of love on the wall of a person's house.   **A** **I**

6. Confide a secret fear.   **A** **I**

7. Put your arm around a person.   **A** **I**

8. Introduce someone to your family.   **A** **I**

9. Be alone together without adult supervision.   **A** **I**

10. Talk about sex.   **A** **I**

© ETR Associates

☐ Self-Check
☐ I read and followed directions.
☐ My work is neat and complete.
☐ This is my best work.

SELF-CHECK

Comprehensive Health for the Middle Grades

---

2. ASSESSING AFFECTIONATE BEHAVIORS

Groups analyze behaviors

Distribute the **Appropriate or Inappropriate Behavior** activity sheet. Divide the class into groups of 4–6. Attempt to get an equal number of boys and girls in each group. Explain the group assignment:

- Complete the activity sheet individually.
- Discuss your responses and your reasons for them as a group.
- Choose a reporter to report to the class any issues on which members of your group strongly disagreed.

Recap group work

As a class, discuss the situations on the activity sheet. Ask reporters to identify the issues on which there was disagreement. Point out that people have different values and norms.

Ongoing Assessment Assess students' ability to identify appropriate or inappropriate behaviors for expressing affection. Because we are all individual, values and norms will differ somewhat. Students should be able to defend their choices for each statement. Encourage respect for differing opinions.

SHARPEN THE SKILL
COMMUNICATION—CLARIFYING NONVERBAL COMMUNICATION

Students can bring in magazine advertisements, photographs or slides that show people demonstrating affection for each other. Ask them to share these items with the class. Classmates can guess the relationship between the individuals (e.g., parent and child, girlfriend and boyfriend), what they might be saying, what they are doing. Discuss the accuracy of the guesses.

✹

3. WHAT DO OUR FAMILIES THINK?

A FAMILY DISCUSSION ACTIVITY

5 minutes

MATERIALS

◆ completed Appropriate or Inappropriate Behavior (1.2), from Activity 2

◆ Talking About Appropriate Behavior (1.3)

HEALTH & SOCIAL STUDIES

Assign a research project on the changes in what was considered appropriate behavior in the past as contrasted with today. For example, students could compare the changes in swimsuits from 100 years ago to today, or research the changes in openly expressing affection. These reports could make historical comparisons or cultural comparisons. Students should draw some conclusions in their reports.

Initiate family activity

Distribute the **Talking About Appropriate Behavior** family letter. Ask students to take it home with the completed **Appropriate or Inappropriate Behavior** activity sheet. Encourage students to discuss their responses with family members.

TALKING ABOUT APPROPRIATE BEHAVIOR `1.3` ABSTINENCE

Name _____   Date _____   Period _____

Dear Family:

Students are beginning a study of abstinence. This study is based on the philosophy that children at this age should not engage in sexual intercourse.

Today in class, students completed an activity sheet on **Appropriate and Inappropriate Behavior**. Your child has brought this activity sheet home to share with you. You may want to discuss the situations with your child. What behaviors do you think are appropriate and inappropriate for expressing affection?

You are your child's most important educator. I encourage you to share your thoughts and feelings with your child. When you disagree on subjects, try to listen to each other's perspective. If you have any questions, please call.

Sincerely,

_____

© ETR Associates

Comprehensive Health for the Middle Grades

---

4. EXPRESSING YOUR AFFECTION

Students identify ways to express affection

Distribute the **Affectionately Yours** activity sheet, and ask students to complete it.

Recap ways to express affection

Discuss students' responses on the activity sheet. Communicating with the other person about the kind of physical contact that is appropriate and acceptable can help avoid "pressure situations" and misunderstandings. Use the **Expressing Affection** *Instant Expert* as background.

Ongoing Assessment Assess students' ability to understand ways to express affection and ways to have fun that do not involve sex. See the **Affectionately Yours** *Key* for examples.

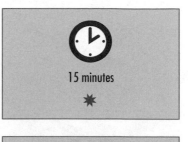

15 minutes

MATERIALS
♦ Affectionately Yours (1.4)

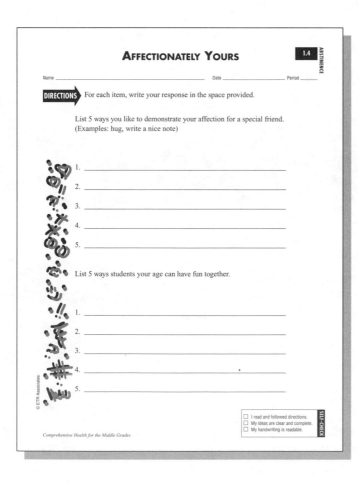

AFFECTIONATELY YOURS   1.4   ABSTINENCE

Name _____ Date _____ Period _____

DIRECTIONS For each item, write your response in the space provided.

List 5 ways you like to demonstrate your affection for a special friend.
(Examples: hug, write a nice note)

1. _____
2. _____
3. _____
4. _____
5. _____

List 5 ways students your age can have fun together.

1. _____
2. _____
3. _____
4. _____
5. _____

☐ I read and followed directions.
☐ My ideas are clear and complete.
☐ My handwriting is readable.
SELF-CHECK

© ETR Associates

Comprehensive Health for the Middle Grades

5. ANY QUESTIONS?

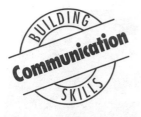

10 minutes

✳

MATERIALS

◆ blank paper

ANONYMOUS QUESTION BOX

◆ shoebox

◆ scissors

✳

Introduce Anonymous Question Box

Display the Anonymous Question Box. Explain that students can use the box to get answers to questions they might be hesitant to ask in class. Provide paper for all students. Students who do not have a question to ask can just write a sentence on the paper to put in the box.

Answer questions

As you teach, be sure to answer students' questions from the Anonymous Question Box. You may want to set up a regular session at the beginning or end of each unit to address these questions.

ANONYMOUS QUESTION BOX

❶ Cut a slit in the lid of a shoebox or other similar box.

❷ Tape the lid to the box.

The box provides the opportunity for all students to get answers to questions they might be hesitant to ask in class. It also gives you time to think about answers to difficult questions or to look for more information.

Tips for Using Anonymous Questions

• Assure students that all questions placed in the box will be taken seriously.

• If you don't know the answer to a question, research it and report back to students.

• Some questions might be better answered privately. Offer students the option of signing their questions if they want a private, written answer.

EVALUATION

OBJECTIVE

Students will be able to:

> **Describe a range of behaviors that demonstrate affection.**

Assess students' responses on the **Affectionately Yours** activity sheet for their ability to describe a range of behaviors that demonstrate affection.

CRITERIA

See the **Affectionately Yours** *Key* for evaluation criteria. Allow students to redo and resubmit if they have not yet achieved the objective.

REVIEW
♦ Affectionately Yours *Key* (p. 14)

MATERIALS
♦ completed Affectionately Yours (1.4), from Activity 4

✳

EXPRESSING AFFECTION

Human beings have many ways to express loving feelings, affection and caring, including gestures, actions, facial expressions and verbal or written comments of appreciation. People can demonstrate affection for others without becoming sexually involved.

Most people feel affection for both men and women. Adolescents who feel affection for peers or adults of the same sex need to know that such feelings are normal. Young people who have concerns about their sexual orientation should be referred for professional counseling.

Feeling attracted to someone does not mean one is in love with that person. Adolescents often confuse feelings of love and desire. Sexual feelings and desires are natural, but they do not have to be acted on.

DEFINING ABSTINENCE

Abstinence from sexual activity means choosing to do without sexual intercourse. People can also abstain from other forms of sexual contact. Abstinence is the only way to provide 100% protection from unintended pregnancy and sexually transmitted disease.

Abstinence is the logical, positive choice for middle school students. At this age, students need time to grow without the emotional upheavals and health risks posed by early sexual relationships. Positive and rewarding friendships are essential at this age; sexual relationships are not.

CULTURAL INFLUENCES ON BEHAVIOR

Culture is the sum total of the way people live, including their beliefs, values and customs. Culture includes the way people express themselves through language—the way they think and communicate—both verbally and nonverbally.

Culture helps determine standards or rules for behavior, called norms. Norms define whether behaviors are appropriate or inappropriate. Values also play an important role in defining appropriateness of behavior. A value is any belief or quality that is important, desirable or prized.

Norms and values define how, when and where it is appropriate and acceptable to express affection. Family members, teachers and friends all play an important role in conveying norms and values. Norms and values vary from culture to culture as well as within cultures.

(continued...)

✱ For more on abstinence, refer to *Abstinence: Health Facts*, pp. 1–10.

EXPRESSING AFFECTION

Values such as respect, self-control and equality can influence decisions about sexual behavior. Students need to be aware of their own values and those of their families, peers, religion, school and community.

PHYSICAL EXPRESSIONS OF AFFECTION

On a continuum, ranging from most to least intimate, some common physical expressions of affection might look like this:

Physical Expressions of Affection

Physical Expressions of Affection

most intimate

sexual intercourse

kissing

arms around shoulders/waist

holding hands

hugging

smiling

least intimate

Preteens and adolescents are very vulnerable to peer pressure. Certain behaviors and settings may be more likely to lead to sexual activity than others. Avoiding the behaviors that are conducive to sexual activity is an important aspect of abstinence.

AFFECTIONATELY YOURS

KEY

 DIRECTIONS For each item, write your response in the space provided.

List 5 ways you like to demonstrate your affection for a special friend. (Examples: hug, write a nice note)

Answers will vary. Examples:

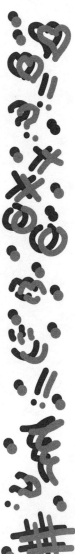

1. **smiling**

2. **holding hands**

3. **arms around shoulders**

4. **giving a gift**

5. **kissing**

List 5 ways students your age can have fun together.

Answers will vary. Examples:

1. **going to a school dance**

2. **going roller skating**

3. **playing miniature golf**

4. **going to an amusement park**

5. **volunteering for a community project**

CRYSTAL BALL

TIME

1–2 periods

ACTIVITIES

1. What Are Your Plans?

2. Pregnancy Changes Your Life

3. Choosing Abstinence

CRYSTAL BALL

Students will be able to:

> Analyze consequences of sexual intercourse for adolescents.

GETTING STARTED

Have:

- *In Your Face* poster *(optional)*

Copy for each student:

- Crystal Ball (2.1)
- Say "Wait" to Sex (2.2)
- Reasons to Wait (2.3)

UNIT OVERVIEW

PURPOSE

Many adolescents have only a vague sense of the future and may not plan beyond the upcoming weekend. They rely on past or present experiences rather than thinking about the future.

Choices students make now can affect them for their entire lives. Encouraging students to look at goals and plans and ways that unplanned pregnancy could interfere with those plans and goals helps them understand the value of abstinence.

MAIN POINTS

✳ Adolescents have many good reasons to choose abstinence.

✳ Unplanned, unanticipated events, such as an unplanned pregnancy, can interfere with goals and plans.

✳ Young people's choices can have life-long effects.

✳ Choosing abstinence now does not preclude having a healthy sexual relationship later.

REVIEW

To increase your understanding of abstinence, review Facts About Abstinence *Instant Expert* (p. 24) and Reasons to Wait *Key* (p. 26).

VOCABULARY

abstain—To refrain from doing something by choice.

abstinence—Avoiding sexual intercourse.

emotions—Feelings about or reactions to certain important events or thoughts.

goal—An end that a person aims to reach or accomplish.

mental/emotional effects—The influence something has on a person's feelings.

plan—A scheme for doing something.

psychological—Having to do with the mind.

risky behaviors—Behaviors that cause an increased likelihood of injury, damage or other negative consequences.

safe—Free from danger.

sexually transmitted disease (STD)—Any of a number of diseases that can spread through sexual contact.

1. WHAT ARE YOUR PLANS?

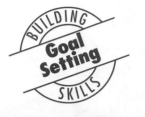

A CLASS DISCUSSION AND SELF-ASSESSMENT ACTIVITY

20 minutes
✴

MATERIALS

◆ Crystal Ball (2.1)
◆ Optional: In Your Face poster
✴

EXTEND THE LEARNING

Display the *In Your Face* poster. Use it as an introduction to these activities related to school-age pregnancy.
✴

Discuss student plans

Ask students what plans they have for the next 6 months. Plans may be personal, social, athletic, academic or school-related. Examples:

- **Personal:** Save money to buy a mountain bike.
- **Social:** Visit my cousin in Canada.
- **Athletic:** Make the basketball team.
- **Academic:** Study hard to get a good report card next semester.
- **School-related:** Join the yearbook staff.

Ask for volunteers to share their plans. Ask students:

- Do your plans always turn out the way you want or expect?
- Are there things you can do to make them more likely to happen?

Students prioritize plans

Distribute the **Crystal Ball** activity sheet. Review the directions and examples. Ask students to list 5 of their plans and prioritize them. Students should write a number from 1 to 5 in the space provided next to each box, with 1 representing the most important plan and 5 representing the least important.

(continued...)

CRYSTAL BALL　2.1　ABSTINENCE

Name _____ Date _____ Period _____

DIRECTIONS ➤ Under the column marked Plans, list 5 things you hope to accomplish or do in the next 6 months. Then rank your plans in order of importance from 1 (most important) to 5 (least important).

Circle any plans that would be affected if you were going to have a baby. Under the column marked Effects, explain how having a baby would affect the plans you circled.

PLANS	EFFECTS
Example: Save money for a mountain bike.	The money will go to baby needs, not the mountain bike.

© ETR Associates

☐ I read and followed directions.
☐ My ideas are clear and complete.
☐ I was honest with myself.
SELF-CHECK

Comprehensive Health for the Middle Grades

---

1. WHAT ARE YOUR PLANS?

CONTINUED

Discuss effects of unplanned pregnancy

Discuss how an unplanned pregnancy might interfere with the example plans on the activity sheet—*Make the basketball team* and *Save money for a mountain bike.* Use the **Facts About Abstinence** *Instant Expert* as a guide. Unanticipated events, such as unplanned pregnancy, can drastically change people's plans.

Students assess plans

Ask students to circle any plans they listed on the activity sheet that would be affected if they were going to have a baby. Then students should explain in the effects column how each of their circled plans might be affected by an unwanted pregnancy.

Ask volunteers to share with the class how an unwanted, unplanned pregnancy would change their personal plans for the next 6 months.

Ongoing Assessment Assess students' ability to identify the effects of an unplanned pregnancy on their plans. For example, buying a mountain bike would be difficult, because any money earned or saved would be needed to support a baby.

SHARPEN THE SKILL
COMMUNICATION—SHARING SENSITIVE INFORMATION

Put students into dyads to roleplay situations where a student must inform another person about a pregnancy. The following are some examples:

- Girlfriend must inform boyfriend that she is pregnant.
- Son must inform a parent that his girlfriend may be pregnant.
- Physician or nurse must inform a teenage girl that she is pregnant.

Make sure each student has the chance to play the communicator. Switch situations around as needed for dyads to conduct the roleplays.

Discuss the experience as a class. Have students talk about how they felt receiving this information as well as sending it. Which was harder? Why?

✳

2. PREGNANCY CHANGES YOUR LIFE

20 minutes

HEALTH & MATH

Statistics: Students can conduct individual or group research projects to gather local statistics on teen pregnancy. They can use math or computer skills to create graphs depicting the statistics.

Groups discuss lifestyle changes

Divide the class into groups of 4–6. Explain the group assignment:

- Discuss possible changes in a young person's life due to pregnancy. Groups should think about changes in themselves, in their relationships (with friends and family), at school and at home.
- Choose a group recorder to record your responses and a reporter to report to the class.

Groups report

Have reporters explain the kinds of changes identified by the group. List the identified changes on the board. Ask students to look at these lists and voice any conclusions they may have.

Ongoing Assessment Students' responses regarding possible lifestyle changes during pregnancy may include:

- changed relationship with parents, friends, boyfriend or girlfriend
- feeling less comfortable with friends
- dropping out of school
- embarrassment
- needing to get a job to support a child

Look for students' understanding that an unplanned pregnancy would affect many aspects of their lives.

3. CHOOSING ABSTINENCE

Discuss STD

Discuss the visible, physical risks of sexual activity, such as sexually transmitted disease (STD). Use the **Facts About Abstinence** *Instant Expert* as a guide. Refraining from sexual activity reduces the risk of contracting STDs such as chlamydia, herpes, gonorrhea and HIV.

Brainstorm other reasons to choose abstinence

Conduct a brainstorming session to identify other reasons for middle school students to choose abstinence. List responses on the board under the heading *"Reasons That Young People Choose Abstinence."* Examples:

- To avoid feelings of guilt, doubt, fear or disappointment.
- Being involved in a sexual relationship can prevent personal growth.
- To avoid disease.
- Religious and moral beliefs.
- Belief that sexual intimacy belongs only in marriage.
- Belief that having sex too soon can hurt a relationship (with partner, parents or others).
- Wanting time to develop deeper friendships—to spend more time talking, building mutual interests and sharing good times.

(continued...)

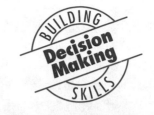

25 minutes

❋

MATERIALS

◆ Say "Wait" to Sex (2.2)

❋

SHARPEN THE SKILL
ASSERTIVENESS—
ARTICULATING
PERSONAL BELIEFS

Making a public declaration of belief is considered an important aspect of establishing healthy behaviors. In the discussion of reasons to choose abstinence, have students use the following lead-in phrase: "I believe it is important to choose abstinence because...."

❋

CONTINUED

MEETING STUDENT NEEDS

Allow students to maintain their privacy on responses on the **Say "Wait" to Sex** activity sheet. Students do not have to write their names on the activity sheet and can keep it for their personal information.

✳

Students identify reasons to wait

Distribute the **Say "Wait" to Sex** activity sheet and ask students to complete it.

Ongoing Assessment Assess students' ability during the brainstorming session to identify reasons to be abstinent. Look for growth in understanding about the consequences of unplanned pregnancy.

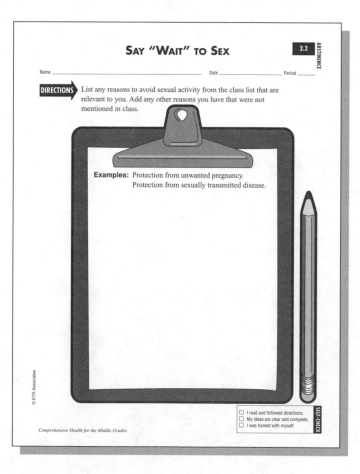

SAY "WAIT" TO SEX 2.2 ABSTINENCE

Name _____ Date _____ Period _____

DIRECTIONS List any reasons to avoid sexual activity from the class list that are relevant to you. Add any other reasons you have that were not mentioned in class.

Examples: Protection from unwanted pregnancy.
Protection from sexually transmitted disease.

☐ I read and followed directions.
☐ My ideas are clear and complete.
☐ I was honest with myself.
SELF-CHECK

© ETR Associates

Comprehensive Health for the Middle Grades

EVALUATION

OBJECTIVE

Students will be able to:

> **Analyze consequences of sexual intercourse for adolescents.**

Distribute the **Reasons to Wait** evaluation sheet. Ask students to complete it by listing the 5 best reasons to wait.

CRITERIA

Assess students' ability to identify reasons to choose abstinence. See the **Reasons to Wait** *Key* for evaluation criteria.

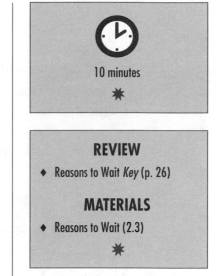

10 minutes

REVIEW

♦ Reasons to Wait *Key* (p. 26)

MATERIALS

♦ Reasons to Wait (2.3)

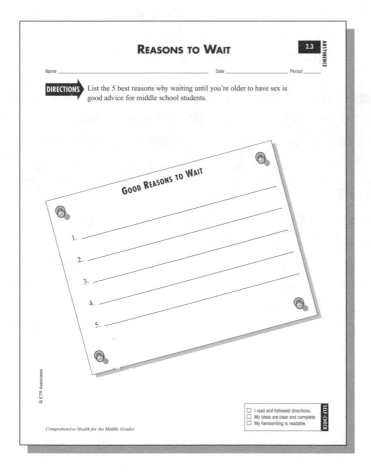

REASONS TO WAIT | 2.3 | ABSTINENCE

Name _____ Date _____ Period _____

DIRECTIONS List the 5 best reasons why waiting until you're older to have sex is good advice for middle school students.

GOOD REASONS TO WAIT

1. _____
2. _____
3. _____
4. _____
5. _____

☐ I read and followed directions.
☐ My ideas are clear and complete.
☐ My handwriting is readable.
SELF-CHECK

© ETR Associates

Comprehensive Health for the Middle Grades

FACTS ABOUT ABSTINENCE

Sex can create problems and concerns in a young person's life. If sexual intercourse contradicts family values or religious beliefs, a young person may experience strong feelings of guilt. Delaying sexual intercourse can be advantageous for several reasons, including:

- avoiding pregnancy
- reducing the risk of contracting sexually transmitted disease (STD), including HIV (the virus that causes AIDS)
- reducing emotional and psychological consequences

PREVENTING PREGNANCY

More than 1 million teenagers get pregnant each year; 80% of these pregnancies are unplanned. Pregnancy can occur the first time a couple has sex. The most obvious reason not to have sex is to reduce the risk of unwanted pregnancy. Abstinence provides 100% protection from pregnancy. All other methods to prevent pregnancy (contraceptive methods) carry a risk of failure.

Unplanned events such as a pregnancy interfere with life goals. Both males and females need to be concerned about such consequences. For females, the consequences include the physical and emotional changes that accompany pregnancy, as well as lifestyle changes.

For males, the consequences may be less obvious, but males face both legal and financial responsibilities for unplanned pregnancy. They may also be affected emotionally. Accepting responsibility for pregnancy may also entail changes in a young man's lifestyle.

REASONS TO CHOOSE ABSTINENCE

Each year in the United States, more than 1 million teenagers become pregnant. U.S. teenagers have 1 of the highest pregnancy rates in the Western World—higher than England, France, Canada, Sweden, the Netherlands and Wales. Yet surveys indicate that many teens in the United States do practice abstinence; 40% of unmarried males and 50% of unmarried females ages 15–19 have never had intercourse.

(continued...)

FACTS ABOUT ABSTINENCE

Personal Reasons

Many young people believe in and practice abstinence because of religious reasons and personal beliefs. Abstinence can be a sign of emotional maturity and integrity. Many young women and men report feeling pressured into having sexual intercourse before they are ready. It requires maturity and honesty to be able to resist pressure from someone you love in order to make a decision that is consistent with personal values, morals and needs.

Medical Reasons

- Abstinence is the only method of birth control that is 100% effective and 100% free of side effects.
- Abstinence reduces the risk of unwanted pregnancy. (Pregnancy can occur without sexual intercourse if sperm is ejaculated near the entrance to the vagina during heavy petting.)
- Abstinence reduces the risk of contracting chlamydia, herpes, gonorrhea and other sexually transmitted disease. (STD can be passed by sexual contact with an infected person.)
- Abstinence reduces the risk of cervical cancer. Cancer researchers are now suggesting a connection between early sexual activity, multiple sexual partners and increased incidence of cervical cancer in women under 25.
- Abstinence is an effective way to decrease the risk of being infected with HIV.

Relationship Reasons

- A couple may find that delaying sexual intercourse contributes in a positive way to their relationship.
- Abstinence may allow a couple time to develop a deeper friendship. They may spend more time talking, building mutual interests, sharing their good times with other friends and establishing an intimacy that is other than sexual.
- Abstinence can be a test of love. Counter to the old line "you would if you loved me," abstinence can allow time to test the endurance of love beyond the first attraction and before having sexual intercourse.
- Abstinence may contribute to teaching a couple to be more loving people and to explore a wide range of ways to express love and sexual feelings.

Key

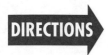

DIRECTIONS List the 5 best reasons why waiting until you're older to have sex is good advice for middle school students.

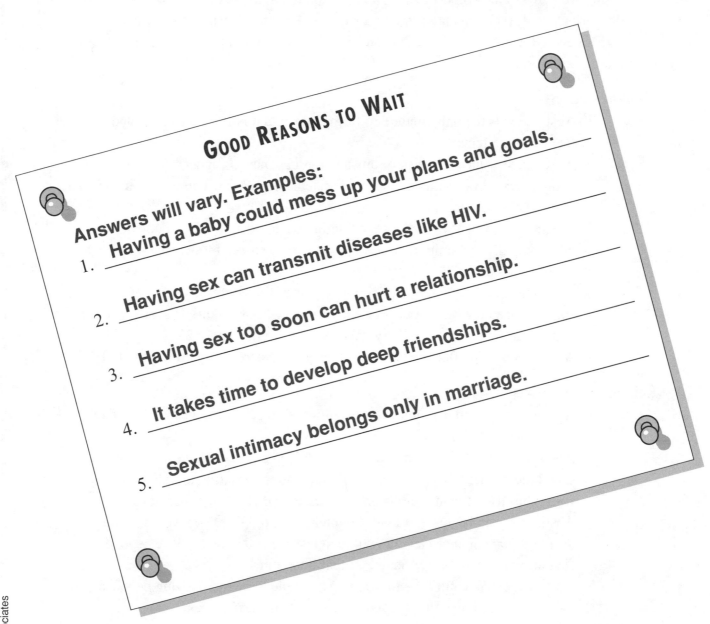

GOOD REASONS TO WAIT

Answers will vary. Examples:

1. Having a baby could mess up your plans and goals.

2. Having sex can transmit diseases like HIV.

3. Having sex too soon can hurt a relationship.

4. It takes time to develop deep friendships.

5. Sexual intimacy belongs only in marriage.

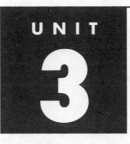

STAYING SAFE

TIME
1–2 periods

ACTIVITIES
1. Is It Safe?
2. Choices and Consequences
3. Family Ideas

STAYING SAFE

OBJECTIVE

Students will be able to:

> Identify uncomfortable situations and settings that may be conducive to sexual behavior.

GETTING STARTED

Have:

- butcher paper or posterboard
- markers
- *Fred and Frieda* poster *(optional)*

Copy 1 for each group:

- Choices and Consequences (3.1)

Copy for each student:

- What My Family Thinks (3.2)
- Sharing Opinions (3.3)

UNIT OVERVIEW

PURPOSE

Young people often face responsibility for sexual behavior before they have reached full emotional and social maturity. Students need to understand that they possess the power to control their own behavior. They themselves are "in charge" and "in control" and are responsible for their own decisions and actions.

MAIN POINTS

* People have the power to control their own behavior; they are responsible for their decisions and actions.
* People need to consider the possible consequences of their decisions and actions.

REVIEW

To increase your understanding of settings and situations that help students remain abstinent, review **Choices and Consequences** *Key* (p. 36).

VOCABULARY

abstinent—Refraining from sexual intercourse by one's own choice.

comfortable—At ease.

consequence—The result of an action.

decision—The result of making up one's mind; a judgment or conclusion.

risky—An increased likelihood of injury, damage or other negative consequences.

safe—Free from danger.

secure—Safe; not worried.

unsafe—Dangerous.

1. Is It Safe?

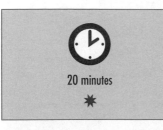

20 minutes

MATERIALS

◆ *Optional: Fred and Frieda poster*

EXTEND THE LEARNING

Display the *Fred and Frieda* poster during this activity. Discuss the "wisdom" and safety of their choices.

Brainstorm uncomfortable situations

Ask students: Have you ever been in a situation where you did not feel comfortable, secure or safe? Conduct a brainstorming session to identify risky situations in which students their age might find themselves. Possible responses:

- going to a dance even though you think you are a horrible dancer
- going to a party where you do not know the other guests
- moving to a new area and going to a new school
- being offered drugs or alcohol at a party
- walking alone at night

Brainstorm safe and unsafe settings

Conduct a brainstorming session to identify safe and unsafe settings for remaining abstinent. Write the headings *"Safe Settings"* and *"Unsafe Settings"* on the board. List students' responses in the appropriate column. Examples:

Safe Settings
- at home with a friend for whom you have romantic feelings while adults are also at home
- a chaperoned party or date

Unsafe Settings
- at home with a friend for whom you have romantic feelings while no adults are home
- an unchaperoned party or date

Brainstorm ways to avoid unsafe settings

Conduct a brainstorming session to identify ways to avoid undesirable and risky situations that might lead to sexual involvement. Examples:

- double dating
- attending only parties that have adult supervision
- spending time only with friends who respect and share your feelings and values

Ongoing Assessment Assess students' ability to identify safe and unsafe settings for choosing to be abstinent and ways to avoid unsafe settings.

2. CHOICES AND CONSEQUENCES

Groups examine case studies

Divide the class into groups of 5. Include both boys and girls in each group. Distribute a copy of the **Choices and Consequences** activity sheet and 3 sheets of butcher paper or posterboard to each group. Explain the group assignment:

- Assign a responsibility to each member—reader, recorder, facilitator, timekeeper, reporter. Rotate group assignments for each case study.
- Read and discuss the case studies.
- Answer the questions about each case study on the activity sheet.
- Copy your choices and the possible consequences for each case study to a piece of butcher paper or posterboard to show the class.
- Decide on the best choice for each situation.
- Prepare a class report. For each case study, explain the choices and consequences and what the group thinks is the best choice and why.

(continued...)

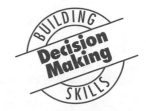

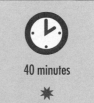

40 minutes

MATERIALS

◆ Choices and Consequences (3.1)
◆ butcher paper or posterboard
◆ markers

MEETING STUDENT NEEDS

Consider your students' maturity level and cultural background before using the **Choices and Consequences** case studies. The acceptable age for dating or attending parties varies widely and is influenced by family and cultural background. Adapt or delete any of the case studies as appropriate for your class.

CHOICES AND CONSEQUENCES

Names _____ Date _____ Period _____

DIRECTIONS ▶ Read each case study. As a group, discuss possible choices for the person. List at least 2 choices. Then discuss and list 2 possible consequences for each choice. Finally, list 1 way to have avoided the situation.

JUANITA'S CASE STUDY

Juanita, an 8th grader, and 2 of her girlfriends went to the local high school hangout on Friday night. Juanita started talking to Carlos, a senior. Carlos invited her to go for a ride in his car. After cruising around town for a few minutes, he stopped the car and put his arm around Juanita.

What are Juanita's choices?
1. _____
_____

2. _____
_____

List 2 consequences of each choice.
1. _____
_____
_____

2. _____
_____
_____

How could the situation have been avoided?
_____
_____

(continued...)

© ETR Associates

Comprehensive Health for the Middle Grades

2. CHOICES AND CONSEQUENCES

SHARPEN THE SKILL

DECISION MAKING— EVALUATING AND MAKING CHANGES

Challenge groups to take the decision making several steps further in their discussions of case studies. Direct them to re-evaluate their choices based on the class discussion and determine the need for any modifications. Groups should provide a brief state-ment that explains any change and the reasoning behind the change.

✴

Groups report

Ask reporters to share the groups' lists of choices and consequences and explain their choices. Discuss the similarities and differences among the choices and consequences listed by different groups.

Ongoing Assessment Observe group reports to assess students' understanding of safe and unsafe settings and situations that may be conducive to sexual behavior. See the **Choices and Consequences** *Key* for assessment criteria. Allow groups to redo and resubmit their work if they have not yet achieved the objective.

3. FAMILY IDEAS

Students interview family members

Distribute the **What My Family Thinks** family activity sheet. Have students answer the first 2 questions in class. They are to interview an adult family member and write the family member's answer to the last 2 questions in the appropriate space.

Distribute the **Sharing Opinions** family letter. Ask students to take the letter home with the activity sheet.

(continued...)

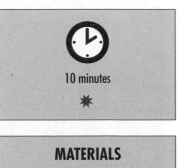

10 minutes

MATERIALS

♦ What My Family Thinks (3.2)
♦ Sharing Opinions (3.3)

WHAT MY FAMILY THINKS | 3.2 | ABSTINENCE

Name _____ Date _____ Period _____

DIRECTIONS Write your answer to the first 2 questions in class. Then take this sheet home and ask an adult family member questions 3 and 4. Write those answers in the space provided.

ASK YOURSELF

1. What are some safe settings and situations for a person my age to be in with a friend for whom I have romantic feelings?

2. What would an adult family member say are some safe settings and situations for a person my age to be in with a friend for whom I have romantic feelings?

ASK AN ADULT

3. What are some safe settings and situations for a person my age to be in with a friend for whom I have romantic feelings?

4. When you were my age, what were considered safe settings and situations to be in with a friend for whom you had romantic feelings?

© ETR Associates

☐ I read and followed directions.
☐ My ideas are clear and complete.
☐ My handwriting is readable.

SELF-CHECK

Comprehensive Health for the Middle Grades

SHARING OPINIONS | 3.3 | ABSTINENCE

Name _____ Date _____ Period _____

Dear Family,

An important part of abstinence is learning to avoid situations that might be conducive to sexual behavior. Examples include:
• being left alone with a special friend with no adults at home
• lying on the couch together to watch TV

Students have an activity sheet, **What My Family Thinks**, to help them identify settings and activities that support abstinence. In class, your child suggested settings he or she thought were safe and predicted what you might say.

The activity sheet has space for your responses. Please discuss with your child the kinds of situations that you consider safe for him or her. If you have any questions, please call.

Sincerely,

_____

© ETR Associates

Comprehensive Health for the Middle Grades

3. FAMILY IDEAS

MEETING STUDENT NEEDS

Be sensitive to the diversity of students' home situations. If students feel uncomfortable with this assignment, modify it to meet their needs. Be sure to respect students' and families' privacy. Students should not be asked to share families' opinions with the class, but only their reactions to the activity.

✳

Discuss family interviews

When students have had time to complete the assignment, discuss the interview process. Ask students:

- Did you enjoy the activity?
- Did this assignment help you talk to adults in your family about your feelings?
- Do you think adult family members can help you deal with some of your questions and problems?

EVALUATION

OBJECTIVE

Students will be able to:

> **Identify uncomfortable situations and settings that may be conducive to sexual behavior.**

Assess students' work in cooperative learning groups and on the **Choices and Consequences** activity sheet for their ability to clearly identify why each situation was uncomfortable and possibly conducive to sexual behavior.

CRITERIA

See the **Choices and Consequences** *Key* for evaluation criteria.

REVIEW

◆ Choices and Consequences *Key* (p. 36)

MATERIALS

◆ completed Choices and Consequences (3.1), from Activity 2

✳

CHOICES AND CONSEQUENCES

KEY

© ETR Associates

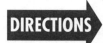 **DIRECTIONS** Read each case study. As a group, discuss possible choices for the person. List at least 2 choices. Then discuss and list 2 possible consequences for each choice. Finally, list 1 way to have avoided the situation.

JUANITA'S CASE STUDY

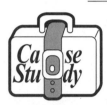 Juanita, an 8th grader, and 2 of her girlfriends went to the local high school hangout on Friday night. Juanita started talking to Carlos, a senior. Carlos invited her to go for a ride in his car. After cruising around town for a few minutes, he stopped the car and put his arm around Juanita.

What are Juanita's choices?

1. **Tell him to keep on driving and to drop her off back at the hangout.**

2. **Say nothing.**

List 2 consequences of each choice.

1. **He will get angry, perhaps drive back recklessly, and not talk to her again.**
   He will respect her feelings, drive back and continue to talk to her.

2. **He could just want to talk and things could be fine.**
   He could start to come on strong, thinking it is OK with her. Then she might have to fight him off later.

How could the situation have been avoided?

If she didn't get into the car alone, she wouldn't have to make either choice.

(continued...)

CHOICES AND CONSEQUENCES

KEY, CONTINUED

JIM'S CASE STUDY

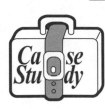

Jim, an 8th grader, was having a Halloween party. The guests, boys and girls from school, were dancing when Jim's mother and father came downstairs to see how the party was going. As soon as Jim's parents left, someone turned off the lights and the room got really dark.

What are Jim's choices?

1. **Turn the lights back on as if it were a joke.**

2. **Do nothing.**

List 2 consequences of each choice.

1. **People would laugh and the party would go on.**
   Jim might get teased.

2. **Things might get out of hand, some people at the party might be uncomfortable.**
   His parents might come down again to check and he would be in a lot of trouble if they found the lights out.

How could the situation have been avoided?
   Let the people coming to the party know what the rules are before they come.

(continued...)

TOM'S CASE STUDY

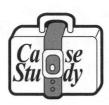

Anita, a 7th grader, invited her boyfriend Tom to her house after school to listen to a new CD. Anita lives with her father but he doesn't get home from work until 8:00 p.m. While they were listening to the music, Anita started kissing Tom.

What are Tom's choices?

1. **Tom could say he needed to go home.**

2. **Tom could kiss her back.**

List 2 consequences of each choice.

1. **Anita could get angry and break up with him.**
   Anita could understand and suggest they go do something else.

2. **They could get more involved than kissing.**
   Anita's dad could show up unexpectedly and call Tom's parents with concerns.

How could the situation have been avoided?
   When Tom found out there was no parent at home he could have suggested they go to his house or do something else.

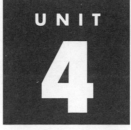

UNIT 4

ASSERTIVE ME!

TIME

2 periods

ACTIVITIES

1. What Is Assertiveness?

2. Are You Assertive?

3. Practice Being Assertive

4. The Assertiveness Log

ASSERTIVE ME!

OBJECTIVE

Students will be able to:

> Demonstrate effective assertive communication skills.

GETTING STARTED

Make transparency of:

- Being Assertive (4.1)

Copy for each student:

- Personal Assertiveness Inventory (4.2)
- Assertiveness Checklist (4.3)
- Assertiveness Log (4.5)

Copy 1 for each group:

- Assertiveness Practice (4.4)

UNIT OVERVIEW

PURPOSE

Most adolescents have a strong need to be part of a group and to be accepted by their peers. Often they do not express their true feelings, needs and opinions because they are afraid of being criticized, chided, unpopular or "different."

This unit focuses on acquiring and practicing assertiveness skills to help students feel confident in expressing their feelings, needs and opinions.

MAIN POINTS

✳ Strong, honest communication is important for successful personal relationships.

✳ Assertiveness skills help people express their feelings, needs and opinions.

REVIEW

To increase your understanding of assertiveness skills, review **Assertiveness Skills** *Instant Expert* (p. 48).

VOCABULARY

assertiveness—Standing up for what one believes, wants or needs, without hurting or denying the rights of others.

aggressiveness—Hostile, demanding, arrogant, pushy, demeaning behavior.

communication—The ability to express thoughts, feelings and reactions and to exchange information.

I-statement—A way to express thoughts, feelings and needs while respecting the rights of others.

1. WHAT IS ASSERTIVENESS?

10 minutes

✳

MATERIALS

♦ Being Assertive (4.1)

✳

Define *assertiveness*

Display the Being Assertive transparency. Ask a student volunteer to read the 2 definitions.

Students identify assertive statements

Ask students: Which of the following statements is assertive?

- You are so stupid! You never invite me to any of your parties.
- I would feel good if you invited me to your party.
- Invite me to your party or you'll be sorry!

Help students distinguish between assertive and aggressive behavior. Aggressive behavior is hostile, demanding, arrogant, pushy, demeaning. Assertive behavior respects both yourself and others.

Review I-statements

One important interpersonal skill is the use of I-statements rather than you-statements. Read the statements again and analyze the difference between them. Explain that I-statements are a good way to respect your own opinions as well as those of others.

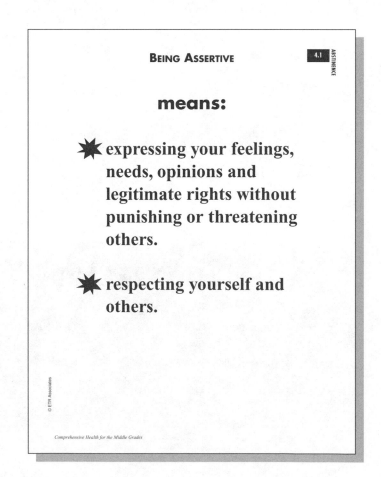

BEING ASSERTIVE   `4.1` ABSTINENCE

means:

✴ **expressing your feelings, needs, opinions and legitimate rights without punishing or threatening others.**

✴ **respecting yourself and others.**

© ETR Associates

Comprehensive Health for the Middle Grades

2. ARE YOU ASSERTIVE?

A SELF-ASSESSMENT ACTIVITY

Students assess assertiveness

Distribute the **Personal Assertiveness Inventory** activity sheet and review the directions. Ask students to complete it. Assure students that this information is for their own knowledge—they do not have to share their responses.

Discuss responses

Ask students to count, for their information only, the number of *always* (A), *sometimes* (S), and *never* (N) responses they marked. More *always* responses indicate they tend to be more assertive; more *never* responses indicate they tend to be less assertive. Practicing assertiveness skills can help them learn to be more assertive.

---

10 minutes
✵

MATERIALS

♦ Personal Assertiveness Inventory (4.2)
✵

MEETING STUDENT NEEDS

Be sensitive to the varying cultural attitudes among your students regarding the concept of assertiveness. In some cultures, direct expression of feelings, needs and opinions is inappropriate.
✵

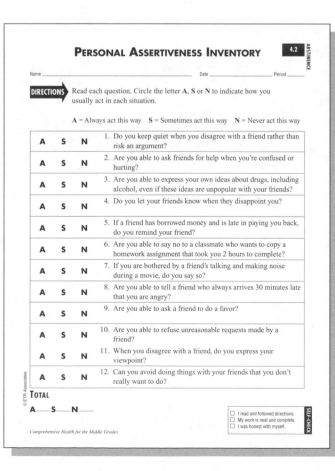

PERSONAL ASSERTIVENESS INVENTORY | 4.2 | ABSTINENCE

Name _____ Date _____ Period _____

DIRECTIONS → Read each question. Circle the letter **A**, **S** or **N** to indicate how you usually act in each situation.

A = Always act this way   **S** = Sometimes act this way   **N** = Never act this way

A S N		1. Do you keep quiet when you disagree with a friend rather than risk an argument?
A S N		2. Are you able to ask friends for help when you're confused or hurting?
A S N		3. Are you able to express your own ideas about drugs, including alcohol, even if these ideas are unpopular with your friends?
A S N		4. Do you let your friends know when they disappoint you?
A S N		5. If a friend has borrowed money and is late in paying you back, do you remind your friend?
A S N		6. Are you able to say no to a classmate who wants to copy a homework assignment that took you 2 hours to complete?
A S N		7. If you are bothered by a friend's talking and making noise during a movie, do you say so?
A S N		8. Are you able to tell a friend who always arrives 30 minutes late that you are angry?
A S N		9. Are you able to ask a friend to do a favor?
A S N		10. Are you able to refuse unreasonable requests made by a friend?
A S N		11. When you disagree with a friend, do you express your viewpoint?
A S N		12. Can you avoid doing things with your friends that you don't really want to do?

TOTAL

A___ **S**___ **N**___

☐ I read and followed directions.
☐ My work is neat and complete.
☐ I was honest with myself.

SELF-CHECK

©ETR Associates

Comprehensive Health for the Middle Grades

---

3. PRACTICE BEING ASSERTIVE

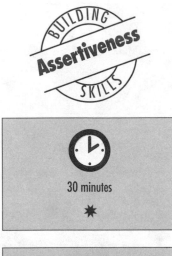

30 minutes

MATERIALS

♦ Assertiveness Checklist (4.3)
♦ Assertiveness Practice (4.4)

Discuss checklist

Distribute the Assertiveness Checklist activity sheet. Discuss how to use the checklist to observe roleplays. Students should use this checklist to assess how assertiveness skills are used during the roleplays they will be observing.

Ask students for examples of I-statements (I want, I need, I feel, I believe) and confident body language (gestures, facial expressions, the way one sits or stands).

Demonstrate roleplays

Ask students to mark their observations on the activity sheet while you demonstrate 2 roleplays. Demonstrate "The Fight" and "The Loan" roleplays, using student volunteers to play Student B. (See page 45.)

After each roleplay, discuss students' observations of Student A (your role). Ask students: How well were feelings, needs, opinions and rights communicated?

(continued...)

ASSERTIVENESS CHECKLIST

4.3

ABSTINENCE

CONTINUED

NAME OF ROLEPLAY: _____
Name of Student A: _____
Name of Student B: _____
Did Student A...
- ✓ Use I-statements? .... Yes   No
- ✓ Insist that Student B hear him or her out? ... Yes   No
- ✓ Use a firm voice? .... Yes   No
- ✓ Use confident body language? .... Yes   No

Observer's Signature: _____

NAME OF ROLEPLAY: _____
Name of Student A: _____
Name of Student B: _____
Did Student A...
- ✓ Use I-statements? .... Yes   No
- ✓ Insist that Student B hear him or her out? ... Yes   No
- ✓ Use a firm voice? .... Yes   No
- ✓ Use confident body language? .... Yes   No

Observer's Signature: _____

NAME OF ROLEPLAY: _____
Name of Student A: _____
Name of Student B: _____
Did Student A...
- ✓ Use I-statements? .... Yes   No
- ✓ Insist that Student B hear him or her out? ... Yes   No
- ✓ Use a firm voice? .... Yes   No
- ✓ Use confident body language? .... Yes   No

Observer's Signature: _____

© ETR Associates

SELF-CHECK
☐ I read and followed directions.
☐ My work is neat and complete.
☐ My handwriting is readable.

Comprehensive Health for the Middle Grades

ASSERTIVENESS PRACTICE

4.4

ABSTINENCE

Name _____   Date _____   Period _____

DIRECTIONS ▶ Roleplay these situations with your group.

1.
MATH HOMEWORK
Student B wants to copy Student A's math homework. Student A spent 2 hours doing this assignment.

2.
AT THE MOVIES
Student A is at the movies with 3 friends. One of the friends, Student B, is talking loudly with a group of boys seated 2 rows behind. Student A can barely hear the dialogue in the movie.

3.
GOING SWIMMING
Student A and Student B agree to meet Saturday morning at 9:00 to catch the bus headed downtown. Student A arrives on time at the bus stop and waits 30 minutes before Student B arrives. This is the second Saturday in a row Student B has arrived late.

4.
CAN YOU COME OVER?
Last night Student A invited a good friend, Student B, to come over. Student B said he or she was sick and needed to stay home and rest. This morning at school Student A learned that Student B was at a dance last night.

© ETR Associates

SELF-CHECK
☐ We did our best work.
☐ Our ideas are clear and complete.
☐ Everyone contributed to the group.

Comprehensive Health for the Middle Grades

---

3. PRACTICE BEING ASSERTIVE

(CONTINUED)

Students practice assertiveness

Divide the class into groups of 4. Distribute the **Assertiveness Practice** activity sheet to each group. Explain the group assignment:

- Take turns roleplaying each of the situations on the activity sheet.
- While 2 students are performing the roleplay, the others act as the observer and the timekeeper.
- The observer should fill out the **Assertiveness Checklist** activity sheet for the roleplay.
- The timekeeper should allow 3 minutes for the roleplay and 1 minute for observer feedback.
- Rotate jobs after each roleplay. Be sure each group member gets to perform each job.

Recap roleplays

Ask volunteers to discuss how easy or difficult it was to assert themselves in each of the roleplay situations. Ask students:

- What was it like to be an observer?
- Was the observer feedback helpful?

Ongoing Assessment Observe students in roleplays and assess their growth in developing assertiveness skills. Specifically look for:

- use of I-statements
- firm voice
- clarification of opinions
- confident posture

SHARPEN THE SKILL

ASSERTIVENESS— RESOLVING CONFLICTS

Have students develop their own conflict situations similar to those demonstrated. Then put them into groups of 4 to act out the plays. Ask a few volunteers to demonstrate for the class.

✳

DEMONSTRATION ROLEPLAYS

Choose a student volunteer to play Student B in each of the following roleplays. You will play the role of Student A, the individual confronted with the difficult situation. Be sure to model effective assertiveness skills.

The Fight
Before leaving for school, Student A had a terrible fight with Mom and is extremely upset. Student A arrives at school and runs into Student B, a good friend. Student A doesn't want to talk with anyone right now.

The Loan
Last month Student A loaned Student B $25. They agreed Student B would pay back the money in a week. Student B still hasn't paid back the loan.

4. THE ASSERTIVENESS LOG

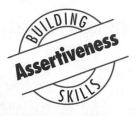

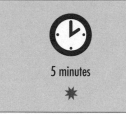

5 minutes

MATERIALS

◆ Assertiveness Log (4.5)

FAMILY LINK

Have students involve family members in their **Assertiveness Log** activity. Students should explain the task and ask family members to help evaluate their progress in appropriate assertive communication. Suggest to students that a good place to start with families is trying to focus on using I-statements rather than you-statements.

Students observe assertiveness skills

Distribute the Assertiveness Log activity sheet. Ask students to track their assertiveness for the next 1–2 days.

Discuss student observations

When students have had time to complete the log, ask volunteers to share their observations. Students should mention people they interacted with by relationship only—friend, brother, parent, teacher—not by name.

Ongoing Assessment Review students' Assertiveness Logs. Look for growth in their ability to:

- identify situations where assertiveness is needed
- analyze their own problems with this skill
- provide appropriate suggestions for improvement

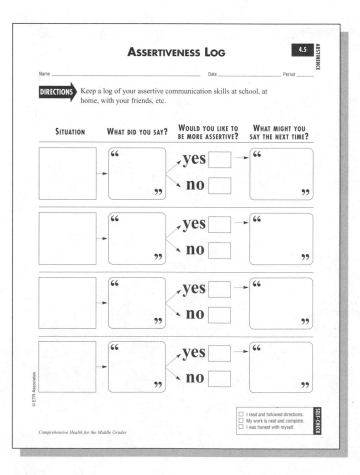

EVALUATION

OBJECTIVE

Students will be able to:

> **Demonstrate effective assertive communication skills.**

Observe students' participation in group roleplays in Activity 3 to assess their ability to demonstrate effective assertive communication skills. Allow students to redo roleplays as necessary.

CRITERIA

Assess student roleplays for:

- use of I-statements
- firm, convincing tone of voice
- confident posture
- clarification of opinions

ASSERTIVENESS SKILLS

Being assertive means being self-respecting. It means being open and honest with yourself as well as with others. It means letting others know you say what you mean and you mean what you say.

Sometimes people hope that others will automatically know what they want, need, feel or believe, but this expectation is rarely met. Strong, honest communication skills are an important component of successful personal relationships.

Assertive people say what they think and stand up for what they believe, want or need without hurting other people or denying their rights. Assertiveness skills help students resist pressures to engage in risky behaviors.

Assertive behavior is not aggressive behavior. Aggression involves overreacting to situations, blaming or criticizing others. Aggression may even involve physical attacks on others.

ASSERTIVENESS SKILLS

Being assertive involves 3 steps:

- stating a position
- offering a reason or explanation
- acknowledging the other person's feelings

I-statements provide an effective technique for assertive communication. An I-statement has 3 parts:

I feel *(describe your feeling)* when you *(describe the behavior),* because *(explain your reason).*

Example: I feel sad when you ignore me, because I want to be your friend.

Other important aspects of assertive communication include:

- using a firm, convincing tone of voice
- confident posture
- clarification of opinions

✱ For more on skills for abstinence, refer to *Abstinence: Health Facts*, pp. 49–57.

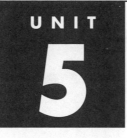

UNIT

5

PRESSURE LINES

TIME

2 periods

ACTIVITIES

1. Saying No to Pressure

2. Practice Saying No

3. What Would You Say?

4. Respecting the Message

5. Positive Self-Talk

PRESSURE LINES

OBJECTIVE

Students will be able to:

> Demonstrate refusal techniques to help them resist pressures to engage in sexual activity.

GETTING STARTED

Have:

- 3" x 5" cards or blank paper

Make transparency of:

- Clearly No (5.1)

Copy for each student:

- Saying No Checklist (5.2)

Copy:

- New CD (5.3), 2–4 copies

Copy 1 for each group:

- At the Mall (5.4)

UNIT OVERVIEW

PURPOSE

Young people need to feel confident they can say no and have it accepted. Refusal techniques are a type of assertive communication that can help students say no to pressures to engage in sexual activity.

MAIN POINTS

✳ Students need to realize that they have the power to control their personal behavior.

✳ Students need to feel confident they can say no and have their refusal accepted.

✳ Practicing refusal techniques helps students feel confident in saying no.

REVIEW

To increase your understanding of refusal techniques, review Learning to Say No *Instant Expert* (p. 61).

VOCABULARY

pressure lines—Statements used to persuade individuals to engage in specific activities.

refusal techniques—Methods of declining or rejecting what is offered.

1. SAYING NO TO PRESSURE

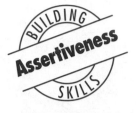

15 minutes

✸

MATERIALS

♦ transparency of Clearly No (5.1)

✸

Discuss pressure lines

Discuss the types of pressure lines young people at this age use to convince others to have sex. Examples:

- Come on, don't be such a baby.
- If you don't want to, I won't see you anymore.
- Everybody's doing it.

Ask students for additional examples.

Discuss ways to say no

Display the Clearly No transparency. Discuss the techniques for saying no. Ask students for examples of the techniques as each one is discussed.

- **Say no and mean it.** There are several ways to show you mean it when you say no.
  - Clearly say the word no.
  - Use a firm voice.
  - Use body language that says no.
  - Refuse to discuss the matter any further.

(continued...)

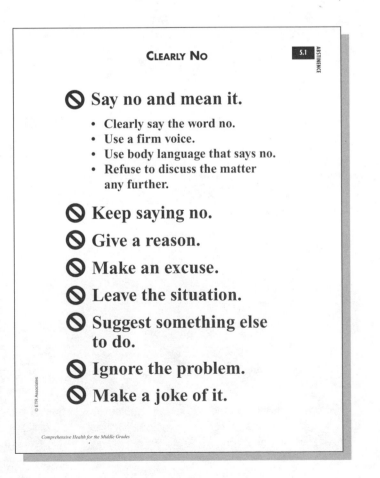

CLEARLY NO   5.1   ABSTINENCE

🚫 **Say no and mean it.**
- Clearly say the word no.
- Use a firm voice.
- Use body language that says no.
- Refuse to discuss the matter any further.

🚫 **Keep saying no.**

🚫 **Give a reason.**

🚫 **Make an excuse.**

🚫 **Leave the situation.**

🚫 **Suggest something else to do.**

🚫 **Ignore the problem.**

🚫 **Make a joke of it.**

© ETR Associates

Comprehensive Health for the Middle Grades

---

1. SAYING NO TO PRESSURE

- **Keep saying no.** This method is sometimes called the "broken record" technique. Continue to say no, without offering excuses or explanations.
- **Give a reason.** Explain why you choose to refuse. For example, if you were pressured to have sex, you might say, "No, I'm not ready to have sex." Ask students for additional examples.
- **Make an excuse.** Examples include: "I have to be home soon," or, "I don't feel well." Ask students for other examples.
- **Leave the situation.** This method can be combined with saying no. Remind students of the unsafe situations discussed in Unit 2.
- **Suggest something else to do.** This is a "delaying tactic." Delaying tactics can help you avoid pressure when it's difficult to say no. Using a delaying tactic doesn't mean you're going to say yes later, but it may give you time to get out of the situation or think of other ways to say no. You can suggest another activity, such as shooting baskets or going to the library. Ask students for other suggestions.
- **Ignore the problem.** This is another delaying tactic. Change the subject or pretend you didn't hear. Ask students for other suggestions.
- **Make a joke of it.** This technique involves using humor. One example is, "If I were ready to have sex, I'd be too old for the 8th grade." Ask students for other examples.

Discuss media influences

Explain that adolescents may also feel pressure from the media. Discuss how the media influences teens to become sexually active. Media influences may include:

- programs on TV
- TV commercials
- songs
- movies or videos
- magazine or newspaper articles and ads

Ask students: As consumers, how might you respond to these influences and pressures from the media?

Discuss pressures (negative positive [handwritten]

SHARPEN THE SKILL
STRESS MANAGEMENT— COPING STRATEGIES

Resisting pressure is stressful. Have students brainstorm a list of coping strategies. Examples:
- exercise
- music
- dancing
- sports
- hobbies

✳

EXTEND THE LEARNING

Have students analyze the messages in current music. The assignment is to find a positive health influence in the music.

Students can bring the lyrics to class and point out the positive messages.

✳

2. PRACTICE SAYING NO

A ROLEPLAY ACTIVITY

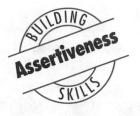

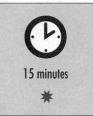

15 minutes

MATERIALS

♦ Saying No Checklist (5.2)

♦ transparency of Clearly No (5.1), from Activity 1

Students assess no-statements

Distribute the Saying No Checklist activity sheet. Discuss how to use the checklist when observing roleplays. Students should use this checklist to assess responses during the roleplays they will be observing.

Demonstrate saying no

Roleplay effective refusal techniques as you say no to the following pressure lines. Ask a different student volunteer to use each of the following pressure lines:

- Come on, don't be such a baby.
- If you don't want to do it, I guess we won't see each other anymore.
- Everybody's doing it!

Use the techniques listed on the **Clearly No** transparency to give clear "no" responses to each of these lines. Ask students to complete the checklist after each roleplay. Discuss their observations. Which techniques did they observe you using?

(continued...)

SAYING NO CHECKLIST   5.2 ABSTINENCE

Name _____ Date _____ Period _____

DIRECTIONS Fill in the pressure line and the names of Student A and Student B for each roleplay you observe. Circle either Yes or No to answer each question. Then sign your name.

PRESSURE LINE: _____

Name of Student A: _____
Name of Student B: _____

Did Student A…

✓ Clearly say the word "no"?	Yes No	✓ Ignore the problem?	Yes No
✓ Use a firm voice?	Yes No	✓ Use humor?	Yes No
✓ Repeat the word "no"?	Yes No	✓ Use body language that said no?	Yes No
✓ Give a reason?	Yes No	✓ Refuse to discuss the matter any further?	Yes No
✓ Suggest something else to do?	Yes No		
✓ Leave the situation?	Yes No		

CONCLUSION

Did Student A use at least 5 refusal techniques?   Yes No
Observer's Signature: _____

PRESSURE LINE: _____

Name of Student A: _____
Name of Student B: _____

Did Student A…

✓ Clearly say the word "no"?	Yes No	✓ Ignore the problem?	Yes No
✓ Use a firm voice?	Yes No	✓ Use humor?	Yes No
✓ Repeat the word "no"?	Yes No	✓ Use body language that said no?	Yes No
✓ Give a reason?	Yes No	✓ Refuse to discuss the matter any further?	Yes No
✓ Suggest something else to do?	Yes No		
✓ Leave the situation?	Yes No		

CONCLUSION

Did Student A use at least 5 refusal techniques?   Yes No
Observer's Signature: _____

(continued...)

Comprehensive Health for the Middle Grades

© ETR Associates

2. PRACTICE SAYING NO

Ongoing Assessment Students should be able to distinguish each of the behaviors on the **Saying No Checklist**. These include:

- clearly saying the word "no"
- using a firm voice
- using body language that says no
- refusing to discuss the matter any further

HEALTH & SCIENCE

Ask students to research the scientific properties of "pressure." If possible, conduct an experiment that demonstrates pressure. Then discuss the relationship to peer pressure.

✳

3. WHAT WOULD YOU SAY?

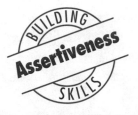

30 minutes

MATERIALS

♦ 3" x 5" cards or blank paper
♦ Saying No Checklist (5.2)

Students list pressure lines

Distribute blank cards or small pieces of paper. Ask students to write 1–2 pressure lines students their age might use to try to convince someone to do something of a sexual nature or to engage in other risky behavior.

Groups roleplay responses

Divide the class into groups of 3. Explain the group assignment:

- Use the pressure lines the members of your group wrote to roleplay saying no to sexual pressures.
- A group member should play the person using a pressure line while another member responds.
- The third member acts as the observer and completes the **Saying No Checklist.**
- After roleplaying a pressure line and a response, switch roles and roleplay the next pressure line.

Recap roleplays

Ask students:

- Were you able to say no in ways that told the other person you meant what you said without losing the friendship?
- Which techniques seemed most effective for saying no?
- Which techniques are you most comfortable using?

Ongoing Assessment Assess students' ability to make clear no-statements, using the described techniques. Allow students to practice and revise their roleplays if they have not yet achieved the objective.

4. Respecting the Message

Discuss respect for others

Ask students:

- Have you ever said no to someone and been ignored?
- What did you do?
- How did you feel?

Explain that an important aspect of respecting ourselves and others is respecting another person's right to say no.

Students read dialogs

Choose 2–4 students to read the **New CD** dialog. Distribute copies of the dialog. Set the stage for the dialog, then have students read Take 1 and then Take 2. Ask the class:

- What is the biggest difference between the dialogs?
- What do you think would happen in Take 1? Would Terry and JJ stay together? Why or why not?

(continued...)

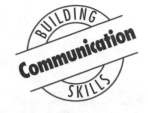

30 minutes

MATERIALS

- New CD (5.3)
- At the Mall (5.4)

NEW CD `5.3` ABSTINENCE

Name _____ Date _____ Period _____

SETTING THE STAGE

JJ and Terry have been going together for several weeks. This weekend, Terry's parents are gone. Terry's cousin is staying at the house with Terry, but has gone out to a movie. Terry is trying to convince JJ to come over.

TAKE 1

Terry: Hey, I have a new CD. Why don't you come over so we can listen to it?

JJ: I thought your parents were out of town this weekend.

Terry: Yeah, they're gone, but my cousin is staying here. Why don't you come over now?

JJ: Is your cousin going to be there?

Terry: No, my cousin went to a movie, so we can be alone. That's OK with you, isn't it?

JJ: Well, I really would like to come over, but I don't think it's a good idea for me to be there when no one else is there.

Terry: Why not? I thought you liked me. I think it would be great to be alone.

JJ: I do like you, but I don't think it's a good idea for me to come over there now.

Terry: What's wrong with you? Nobody else would have a problem with it. You're not afraid of me, are you?

JJ: No.

Terry: Then come on over.

JJ: Well....

(continued...)

© ETR Associates

Comprehensive Health for the Middle Grades

4. Respecting the Message

Groups write dialogs

Divide the class into groups of 3–4. Distribute the **At the Mall** activity sheet to each group. Explain the group assignment:

- Use this setting or create a new one to write a dialog about someone saying no to a friend's pressure to do something risky.
- Write 2 endings for the dialog. The first ending should show what happens if the friend doesn't respect the no response; the second ending should show respect for the response.
- Decide who will read which parts of the dialog to the class.

Groups present dialogs

Ask groups to present their dialogs. Discuss the refusal techniques used and how the endings demonstrate the importance of respecting other people's right to say no.

Ongoing Assessment   Look for students' understanding that respecting others' right to say no can help prevent risky situations.

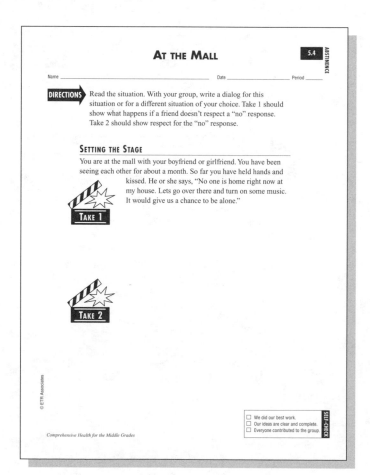

5. POSITIVE SELF-TALK

Brainstorm positive messages

Conduct a brainstorming session to identify positive messages that would support students in saying no to sex. List student suggestions on the board. Ask students to copy this list for their personal reference.

Students create positive statements

Ask students to create a positive self-talk statement for each of the following negative statements:

- If I say no, he'll get another girlfriend.
  Example: I feel good about my decision to say no.
- My friends will tease me if I don't do anything with her.
  Example: We are having a good time together without having sex.

10 minutes

HEALTH & ART

Have students create posters that have positive messages for teens that support the choice to abstain.

EVALUATION

OBJECTIVE

Students will be able to:

> **Demonstrate refusal techniques to help them resist pressures to engage in sexual activity.**

Observe students' ability to make clear no statements to pressure lines during the roleplay exercises in Activities 3 and 4.

CRITERIA

Look for students to use at least 5 of the following refusal techniques:

- clearly saying the word *no*—using a firm voice and body language that says no and refusing further discussion
- repeating the word *no*
- giving a reason
- making an excuse
- leaving the situation
- suggesting something else to do
- ignoring the problem
- using humor

Learning to Say No

Reasoning, self-discipline, a sense of responsibility, self-control and ethical considerations, such as respect for oneself and others, form a foundation for healthful and safe personal behaviors. People who respect themselves and others are able to resist pressure and do not try to pressure others into actions they don't want to take.

Clear communication promotes understanding of others' feelings and viewpoints. Students can learn techniques that help them say no and resist pressure. The ability to say no gives people power in their lives.

Listening is also an important communication skill. Students need to listen to others' messages and respect their right to say no.

REFUSAL TECHNIQUES

Good refusal techniques clearly say no in a way that leaves no doubt about the intent but doesn't jeopardize the relationship. They can be both verbal and nonverbal. However, there is no good substitute for the word *no*.

A clear no-statement has the following characteristics:
- the word *no*
- a strong nonverbal no
- a repeat of the message as needed
- firm tone of voice

Other ways to say no include:
- giving a reason or an excuse
- suggesting an alternative
- ignoring the problem
- using humor
- leaving the situation

In addition to leaving a pressure situation, other nonverbal refusal techniques include:
- *hands-off hands*—throwing up hands in a "get off of me" gesture or using hands for emphasis
- *soldier body*—sitting or standing stiffly, like a soldier at attention, and marching away if needed
- *serious expression*—a face that says "I mean it"
- *other gestures*—hand and arm movements that emphasize the point
- *fighting back*—if all else fails, pushing away

(continued...)

LEARNING TO SAY NO

SAYING NO TO SEXUAL HARASSMENT AND DATE RAPE

Sexual harassment is unwelcome verbal or physical conduct of a sexual nature. The harassment often involves a person with power over another, but fellow students and coworkers can also be guilty of harassment.

Both boys and girls need to know that they have a right to say no to unwelcome sexual advances and behaviors of a sexual nature with which they feel uncomfortable. The perception of harassment is in the eye of the beholder. If the behavior is unwanted by the recipient, it can be considered harassment.

Date rape, or acquaintance rape, is rape committed by someone the victim knows. Women are more likely to be raped by someone they know than by a stranger. Women (and men) always have the right to say no to sex. However, in American society, men, especially, are not always taught to respect a woman's right to say no. Clear communication and respect for others' feelings can help prevent date rape and sexual harassment.

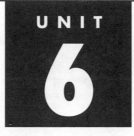

UNIT
6

WE'RE THERE FOR YOU

TIME
1 period

ACTIVITIES
1. Who Supports You?
2. Personal Support Systems
3. Peer Power

WE'RE THERE FOR YOU

OBJECTIVE

Students will be able to:

Identify personal support systems to help them abstain from sex.

GETTING STARTED

Have:

- *Myth and Fact* poster *(optional)*

Copy for each student:

- My Personal Support System (6.1)
- Peer Power Contract (6.2)

UNIT OVERVIEW

PURPOSE

Adolescents, like all people, want to know and feel that the significant people in their lives love and accept them. Personal support systems can help enhance students' self-esteem and help them avoid sexual involvement.

High self-esteem allows people to feel good about themselves and to make positive choices about personal behavior. High self-esteem helps reduce students' vulnerability to pressures from peers and the media to be sexually active. It gives students more power to accomplish their plans and goals.

MAIN POINTS

✳ Personal support systems can help people deal with the difficult situations they confront throughout their lives.

✳ High self-esteem increases self-confidence and helps people make positive choices about behavior.

REVIEW

To increase your understanding of personal support systems and self-esteem, review **Personal Support Systems** *Instant Expert* (p. 71).

VOCABULARY

contract—An agreement between 2 or more people to do something.

peer power—Friends talking friends into doing something positive.

peer pressure—The influence of friends on behavior.

personal support system—Individuals who provide help.

self-esteem—Measure of how much a person values himself or herself.

values—Important beliefs or qualities.

1. WHO SUPPORTS YOU?

10 minutes

✳

MATERIALS

♦ *Optional: Myth and Fact* poster

✳

EXTEND THE LEARNING

Display the *Myth and Fact* poster. Read it aloud to students. Explain that an important part of personal support is knowing that you are not alone in your beliefs. Discuss the fact that abstinence is the choice most middle school students make.

✳

Define personal support system

Write the words PERSONAL SUPPORT SYSTEM on the board. Ask students to think of a difficult time in their lives (death in the family, moving, saying no to drugs, parental separation or divorce). They most likely needed to have a lot of support or help from people who cared about them. The people who helped them are part of their personal support system.

Discuss the concept of personal support systems. Emphasize that the use of a support system is an excellent stress management technique. Use the Personal Support System *Instant Expert* as a guide to this discussion.

Students identify personal support systems

Ask students to name some of the relationships that are part of their personal support systems (friend, aunt or uncle, parent, grandparent, teacher). Caution students not to say names, but just the relationships. List their responses on the board. Discuss how these individuals help them.

Ongoing Assessment   Look for student understanding that we all need people who care about us in times of difficulty or stress.

2. PERSONAL SUPPORT SYSTEMS

A DYAD DISCUSSION ACTIVITY

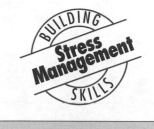

Dyads discuss support systems

Distribute the **My Personal Support System** activity sheet. Ask students to complete it individually. Then have students pair up and discuss their responses.

Discuss access to support systems

Ask students:

- How can you reach out to the people in your personal support system when you have questions about sex? (by telephone, meeting in person, making an appointment)
- What kinds of support people have factual information about sex?
- Do you know when these people are available to talk to you?
- Where can you contact them?
- Can they be trusted to keep your discussions confidential?
- Would you contact this support system if you were tempted to engage in sex?
- If not, why not? How can you identify people you could talk to?

(continued...)

15 minutes

MATERIALS

- My Personal Support System (6.1)

MY PERSONAL SUPPORT SYSTEM — 6.1 ABSTINENCE

Name _____ Date _____ Period _____

DIRECTIONS Write the names and relationships to you of people who can help you abstain from sexual activity. You can list the same person more than once.

For Gathering Information About Sex

Name   Relationship to me

1. _____
2. _____
3. _____

For Talking About Sex

Name   Relationship to me

1. _____
2. _____
3. _____

© ETR Associates

☐ I read and followed directions.
☐ My handwriting is readable.
☐ I was honest with myself.

SELF-CHECK

Comprehensive Health for the Middle Grades

2. PERSONAL SUPPORT SYSTEMS

COMMUNITY LINK

Have students research the places in the community where students their age can get assistance. These may include churches, synagogues, clinics and family counseling centers. Create a poster with phone numbers and locations for these community resources.

✳

Draw conclusions

Have students draw conclusions about the kinds of people who can help. Ask students: What qualities would a good support person have?

Ongoing Assessment Look for students to indicate qualities such as:

- knowledgeable (probably not someone the same age)
- trustworthy
- respectful
- has similar values
- able to listen and share feelings
- able to help solve problems

3. PEER POWER

Discuss peer power

Discuss peer pressure and peer power, using the **Identifying Personal Support Systems** *Instant Expert* as a guide. Ask students:

* What is peer pressure? (the influence of friends on behavior)
* Have you ever heard of peer power?
* What do you think peer power might be? (the positive influence of friends)

Students sign contracts

Distribute the **Peer Power Contract** activity sheet. Ask students to identify a friend who will support their decision to abstain from sexual activity. Friends can sign these contracts for each other. Assure students that the contracts are confidential. Students do not have to share them in class.

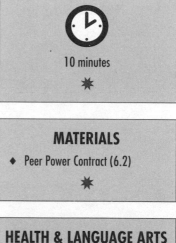

10 minutes

MATERIALS

◆ Peer Power Contract (6.2)

HEALTH & LANGUAGE ARTS

Define the word *contract*. Students should look up the definition, then identify key concepts associated with a contract.

Post the definition and key concepts in the classroom.

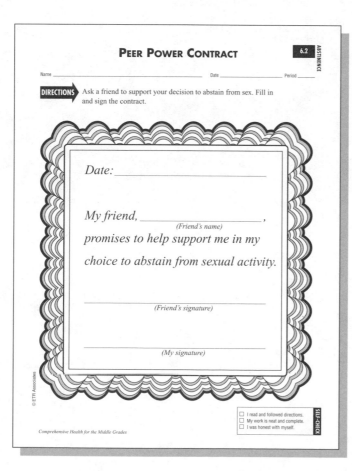

PEER POWER CONTRACT   6.2   ABSTINENCE

Name _____ Date _____ Period _____

DIRECTIONS Ask a friend to support your decision to abstain from sex. Fill in and sign the contract.

Date: _____

My friend, _____,
        (Friend's name)
promises to help support me in my choice to abstain from sexual activity.

_____
(Friend's signature)

_____
(My signature)

© ETR Associates

Comprehensive Health for the Middle Grades

☐ I read and followed directions.
☐ My work is neat and complete.
☐ I was honest with myself.   SELF-CHECK

EVALUATION

OBJECTIVE

Students will be able to:

> **Identify personal support systems to help them abstain from sex.**

Ask students to review the people they identified on the **My Personal Support System** activity sheet and think about any changes they may want to make based on what they have learned. Have students identify another list of people for their support system, then write a paragraph explaining why they did or did not change the list from the original one on the activity sheet.

CRITERIA

Assess students' ability to identify people who can support them to abstain from sex. Look for paragraphs to identify qualities such as:

- knows the facts or where to get the facts
- trustworthy
- able to listen and share feelings
- respectful
- has similar values
- can help solve problems

PERSONAL SUPPORT SYSTEMS

Middle school students may have many unanswered questions about sex. They may be unsure of the facts and of their own feelings and values. A personal support system can help students sort out their thoughts and feelings. It is an excellent way to deal with stress.

At different times, students may want or need to talk with parents or other trusted, supportive adults about personal thoughts and feelings. In their search for understanding and support, they often decide to talk to friends and siblings as well.

The appropriate people to talk to might be determined by the information students are seeking. Some general kinds of information-seeking include:

- gathering facts
- sharing feelings
- exploring values
- making decisions

Effective support people will perform some or all of the following tasks:

- listening as thoughts and feelings are shared
- helping to sort out facts
- discussing possible actions

PEER PRESSURE OR PEER POWER

Peer pressure refers to the influence, either physical or mental, of friends on behavior. Peer pressure can be either negative or positive. Positive peer pressure can be called "peer power."

Peer power encourages students to make healthy choices, such as refraining from tobacco, alcohol and other drug use, and abstaining from sexual activity. It's an aspect of setting up social norms that support healthy behaviors.

ENHANCING SELF-ESTEEM

The way others see us can affect our self-esteem or the way we feel about ourselves. If others see us in a positive light, we tend to appreciate our own personal qualities even more.

Personal support is an important factor related to resiliency—the ability to cope with problems and accept ourselves as we are. Resilient people may experience stress, frustration and feelings of self-doubt or failure, but they are able to recapture a sense of mental wellness within a reasonable period of time. People with high self-esteem are resilient.

Students with enhanced self-esteem feel more self-confident. This self-esteem and self-confidence can help students resist peer pressure to engage in sexual activity.

✴ For more on influences on the choice to abstain, refer to *Abstinence: Health Facts,* pp. 39–47.

FINAL
EVALUATION

FINAL EVALUATION

Evaluate student learning

For the final evaluation, students create a culminating project that demonstrates their choice to be abstinent.

Ask students to work individually or in small groups to create a dialog, play, poster or other creative piece that clearly demonstrates the choice to be abstinent.

Ask students to use at least 2 of the following concepts and skills:

- assertive communication skills
- refusal techniques
- avoiding situations and settings that might be conducive to sexual behavior
- personal support systems
- positive self-talk
- respect for others' refusals

CRITERIA

Projects should demonstrate the choice to be abstinent. Assess students' use of at least 2 of the concepts and skills taught. Examples:

- effective communication skills
- effective refusal techniques
- avoidance of risky situations
- the use of personal support systems
- positive self-talk
- respect for others' refusals

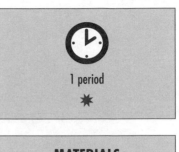

1 period
✳

MATERIALS

♦ *Optional:* art supplies
✳

COMMUNITY LINK

Students can present their dialogs or plays at a school assembly or home and school club meeting. If you have access to a video recorder, students' pieces can be recorded for presentation to other classes and/or community groups. Be sure to assess appropriateness of the programs for presentation to other groups.

✳

APPENDIXES

Why Comprehensive School Health?

Components of a
Comprehensive Health Program

The Teacher's Role

Teaching Strategies

Glossary

Resources and References

WHY COMPREHENSIVE SCHOOL HEALTH?

The quality of life we ultimately achieve is determined in large part by the health decisions we make, the subsequent behaviors we adopt, and the public policies that promote and support the establishment of healthy behaviors.

A healthy student is capable of growing and learning; of producing new knowledge and ideas; of sharing, interacting and living peacefully with others in a complex and changing society. Fostering healthy children is the shared responsibility of families, communities and schools.

Health behaviors, the most important predictors of current and future health status, are influenced by a variety of factors. Factors that lead to and support the establishment of healthy behaviors include:

- awareness and knowledge of health issues
- the skills necessary to practice healthy behaviors
- opportunities to practice healthy behaviors
- support and reinforcement for the practice of healthy behaviors

The perception that a particular healthy behavior is worthwhile often results in young people becoming advocates, encouraging others to adopt the healthy behavior. When these young advocates exert pressure on peers to adopt healthy behaviors, a healthy social norm is established (e.g., tobacco use is unacceptable in this school).

Because health behaviors are learned, they can be shaped and changed. Partnerships between family members, community leaders, teachers and school leaders are a vital key to the initial development and maintenance of children's healthy behaviors and can also play a role in the modification of unhealthy behaviors. Schools, perhaps more than any other single agency in our society, have the opportunity to influence factors that shape the future health and productivity of Americans.

When young people receive reinforcement for the practice of a healthy behavior, they feel good about the healthy behavior. Reinforcement and the subsequent good feeling increase the likelihood that an individual will continue to practice a behavior and thereby establish a positive health habit. The good feeling and the experience of success motivate young people to place a high value on the behavior (e.g., being a nonsmoker is good).

From *Step by Step to Comprehensive School Health,* W. M. Kane (Santa Cruz, CA: ETR Associates, 1992).

Components of a Comprehensive Health Program

The school's role in fostering the development of healthy students involves more than providing classes in health. There are 8 components of a comprehensive health education program:

- **School Health Instruction**—Instruction is the in-class aspect of the program. As in other subject areas, a scope of content defines the field. Application of classroom instruction to real life situations is critical.

- **Healthy School Environment**—The school environment includes both the physical and psychological surroundings of students, faculty and staff. The physical environment should be free of hazards; the psychological environment should foster healthy development.

- **School Health Services**—School health services offer a variety of activities that address the health status of students and staff.

- **Physical Education and Fitness**—Participation in physical education and fitness activities promotes healthy development. Students need information about how and why to be active and encouragement to develop skills that will contribute to fitness throughout their lives.

- **School Nutrition and Food Services**—The school's nutritional program provides an excellent opportunity to model healthy behaviors. Schools that provide healthy food choices and discourage availability of unhealthy foods send a clear message to students about the importance of good nutrition.

- **School-Based Counseling and Personal Support**—School counseling and support services play an important role in responding to special needs and providing personal support for individual students, teachers and staff. These services can also provide programs that promote schoolwide mental, emotional and social well-being.

- **Schoolsite Health Promotion**—Health promotion is a combination of educational, organizational and environmental activities designed to encourage students and staff to adopt healthier lifestyles and become better consumers of health care services. It views the school and its activities as a total environment.

- **School, Family and Community Health Promotion Partnerships**—Partnerships that unite schools, families and communities can address communitywide issues. These collaborative partnerships are the cornerstone of health promotion and disease prevention.

THE TEACHER'S ROLE

The teacher plays a critical role in meeting the challenge to empower students with the knowledge, skills and ability to make healthy behavior choices throughout their lives.

Instruction

Teachers need to provide students with learning opportunities that go beyond knowledge. Instruction must include the chance to practice skills that will help students make healthy decisions.

Involve Families and Communities

The issues in health are real-life issues, issues that families and communities deal with daily. Students need to see the relationship of what they learn at school to what occurs in their homes and their communities.

Model Healthy Behavior

Teachers educate students by their actions too. Students watch the way teachers manage health issues in their own lives. Teachers need to ask themselves if they are modeling the health behaviors they want students to adopt.

Maintain a Healthy Environment

The classroom environment has both physical and emotional aspects. It is the teacher's role to maintain a safe physical environment. It is also critical to provide an environment that is sensitive, respectful and developmentally appropriate.

Establish Groundrules

It is very important to establish classroom groundrules before discussing sensitive topics or issues. Setting and consistently enforcing groundrules establishes an atmosphere of respect, in which students can share and explore their personal thoughts, feelings, opinions and values.

Refer Students to Appropriate Services

Teachers may be the first to notice illness, learning disorders or emotional distress in students. The role of the teacher is one of referral. Most districts have guidelines for teachers to follow.

Legal Compliance

Teachers must make every effort to communicate to parents and other family members about the nature of the curriculum. Instruction about certain topics, such as sexuality, HIV or drug use, often must follow notification guidelines regulated by state law. Most states also require teachers to report any suspected cases of child abuse or neglect.

TEACHING STRATEGIES

The resource books incorporate a variety of instructional strategies. This variety is essential in addressing the needs of different kinds of learners. Different strategies are grouped according to their general education purpose. When sequenced, these strategies are designed to help students acquire the knowledge and skills they need to choose healthy behavior. Strategies are identified with each activity. Some strategies are traditional, while others are more interactive, encouraging students to help each other learn.

The strategies are divided into 4 categories according to their general purpose:

- providing key information
- encouraging creative expression
- sharing thoughts, feelings and opinions
- developing critical thinking

The following list details strategies in each category.

Providing Key Information

Information provides the foundation for learning. Before students can move to higher-level thinking, they need to have information about a topic. In lieu of a textbook, this series uses a variety of strategies to provide students the information they need to take actions for their health.

Anonymous Question Box

An anonymous question box provides the opportunity for all students to get answers to questions they might be hesitant to ask in class. It also gives teachers time to think about answers to difficult questions or to look for more information.

Questions should be reviewed and responded to regularly, and all questions placed in the box should be taken seriously. If you don't know the answer to a question, research it and report back to students.

You may feel that some questions would be better answered privately. Offer students the option of signing their questions if they want a private, written answer. Any questions not answered in class can then be answered privately.

Current Events

Analyzing local, state, national and international current events helps students relate classroom discussion to everyday life. It also helps students understand how local, national and global events and policies affect health status. Resources for current events include newspapers, magazines and other periodicals, radio and television programs and news.

Demonstrations and Experiments

Teachers, guest speakers or students can use demonstrations and experiments to show how something works or why something is important. These activities also provide a way to show the correct process for doing something, such as a first-aid procedure.

Demonstrations and experiments should be carefully planned and conducted. They often involve the use of supporting materials.

Games and Puzzles

Games and puzzles can be used to provide a different environment in which learning can take place. They are frequently amusing and sometimes competitive.

Many types of games and puzzles can be adapted to present and review health concepts. It may be a simple question-and-answer game or an adaptation of games such as Bingo, Concentration or Jeopardy. Puzzles include crosswords and word searches.

A game is played according to a specific set of rules. Game rules should be clear and simple. Using groups of students in teams rather than individual contestants helps involve the entire class.

Guest Speakers

Guest speakers can be recruited from students' families, the school and the community. They provide a valuable link between the classroom and the "real world."

Speakers should be screened before being invited to present to the class. They should have some awareness of the level of student knowledge and should be given direction for the content and focus of the presentation.

Interviewing

Students can interview experts and others about a specific topic either inside or outside of class. Invite experts, family members and others to visit class, or ask students to interview others (family members or friends) outside of class.

Advance preparation for an organized interview session increases the learning potential. A brainstorming session before the interview allows students to develop questions to ask during the interview.

TEACHING STRATEGIES

Oral Presentations

Individual students or groups or panels of students can present information orally to the rest of the class. Such presentations may sometimes involve the use of charts or posters to augment the presentation.

Students enjoy learning and hearing from each other, and the experience stimulates positive interaction. It also helps build students' communication skills.

Encouraging Creative Expression

Student creativity should be encouraged and challenged. Creative expression provides the opportunity to integrate language arts, fine arts and personal experience into a lesson. It also helps meet the diverse needs of students with different learning styles.

Artistic Expression or Creative Writing

Students may be offered a choice of expressing themselves in art or through writing. They may write short stories, poems or letters, or create pictures or collages about topics they are studying. Such a choice accommodates the differing needs and talents of students.

This technique can be used as a follow-up to most lessons. Completed work should be displayed in the classroom, at school or in the community.

Dramatic Presentations

Dramatic presentations may take the form of skits or mock news, radio or television shows. They can be presented to the class or to larger groups in the school or community. When equipment is available, videotapes of these presentations provide an opportunity to present students' work to other classes in the school and other groups in the community.

Such presentations are highly motivating activities, because they actively involve students in learning desired concepts. They also allow students to practice new behaviors in a safe setting and help them personalize information presented in class.

Roleplays

Acting out difficult situations provides students practice in new behaviors in a safe setting. Sometimes students are given a part to play, and other times they are given an idea and asked to improvise. Students need time to decide the central action of the situation and how they will resolve it before they make their presentation. Such activities are highly motivating because they actively involve students in learning desired concepts or practicing certain behaviors.

Sharing Thoughts, Feelings and Opinions

In the sensitive areas of health education, students may have a variety of opinions and feelings. Providing a safe atmosphere in which to discuss opinions and feelings encourages students to share their ideas and listen and learn from others. Such discussion also provides an opportunity to clarify misinformation and correct misconceptions.

Brainstorming

Brainstorming is used to stimulate discussion of an issue or topic. It can be done with the whole class or in smaller groups. It can be used both to gather information and to share thoughts and opinions.

All statements should be accepted without comment or judgment from the teacher or other students. Ideas can be listed on the board, on butcher paper or newsprint or on a transparency. Brainstorming should continue until all ideas have been exhausted or a predetermined time limit has been reached.

Class Discussion

A class discussion led by the teacher or by students is a valuable educational strategy. It can be used to initiate, amplify or summarize a lesson. Such discussions also provide a way to share ideas, opinions and concerns that may have been generated in small group work.

Clustering

Clustering is a simple visual technique that involves diagraming ideas around a main topic. The main topic is written on the board and circled. Other related ideas are then attached to the central idea or to each other with connecting lines.

Clustering can be used as an adjunct to brainstorming. Because there is no predetermined number of secondary ideas, clustering can accommodate all brainstorming ideas.

Continuum Voting

Continuum voting is a stimulating discussion technique. Students express the extent to which they agree or disagree with a statement read by the teacher. The classroom should be prepared for this activity with a sign that says "Agree" on one wall and a sign that says "Disagree" on the opposite wall. There should be room for students to move freely between the 2 signs.

As the teacher reads a statement, students move to a point between the signs that reflects their thoughts or feelings. The closer to the "Agree" sign they stand, the stronger their agreement. The closer to the "Disagree" sign they stand, the stronger their disagreement. A position in the center between the signs indicates a neutral stance.

Dyad Discussion

Working in pairs allows students to provide encouragement and support to each other. Students who may feel uncomfortable sharing in the full class may be more willing to share their thoughts and feelings with 1 other person. Depending on the task, dyads may be temporary, or students may meet regularly with a partner and work together to achieve their goals.

Forced Field Analysis

This strategy is used to discuss an issue that is open to debate. Students analyze a situation likely to be approved by some students and opposed by others. For example, if the subject of discussion was the American diet, some students might support the notion that Americans consume healthy foods because of the wide variety of foods available. Other students might express concern about the amount of foods that are high in sodium, fat and sugar.

Questioning skills are critical to the success of this technique. A good way to open such a discussion is to ask students, "What questions should you ask to determine if you support or oppose this idea?" The pros and cons of students' analysis can be charted on the board or on a transparency.

Journal Writing

Journal writing affords the opportunity for thinking and writing. Expressive writing requires that students become actively involved in the learning process. However, writing may become a less effective tool for learning if students must worry about spelling and punctuation. Students should be encouraged to write freely in their journals, without fear of evaluation.

Panel Discussion

Panel discussions provide an opportunity to discuss different points of view about a health topic, problem or issue. Students can research and develop supporting arguments for different sides. Such research and discussion enhances understanding of content.

Panel members may include experts from the community as well as students. Panel discussions are usually directed by a moderator and may be followed by a question and answer period.

Self-Assessment

Personal inventories provide a tool for self-assessment. Providing privacy around personal assessments allows students to be honest in their responses. Volunteers can share answers or the questions can be discussed in general, but no students should have to share answers they would prefer to keep private. Students can use the information to set personal goals for changing behaviors.

Small Groups

Students working together can help stimulate each other's creativity. Small group activities are cooperative, but have less formal structure than cooperative learning groups. These activities encourage collective thinking and provide opportunities for students to work with others and increase social skills.

Surveys and Inventories

Surveys and inventories can be used to assess knowledge, attitudes, beliefs and practices. These instruments can be used to gather knowledge about a variety of groups, including students, parents and other family members, and teachers.

Students can use surveys others have designed or design their own. When computers are available, students can use them to summarize their information, create graphs and prepare presentations of the data.

Developing Critical Thinking

Critical thinking skills help students analyze health topics and issues. These activities require that students learn to gather information, consider the consequences of actions and behaviors and make responsible decisions. They challenge students to perform higher-level thinking and clearly communicate their ideas.

Case Studies

Case studies provide written histories of a problem or situation. Students can read, discuss and analyze these situations. This strategy encourages student involvement and helps students personalize the health-related concepts presented in class.

Teaching Strategies

Cooperative Learning Groups

Cooperative learning is an effective teaching strategy that has been shown to have a positive effect on students' achievement and interpersonal skills. Students can work in small groups to disseminate and share information, analyze ideas or solve problems. The size of the group depends on the nature of the lesson and the make-up of the class. Groups work best with from 2–6 members.

Group structure will affect the success of the lessons. Groups can be formed by student choice, random selection, or a more formal, teacher-influenced process. Groups seem to function best when they represent the variety and balance found in the classroom. Groups also work better when each student has a responsibility within the group (reader, recorder, timer, reporter, etc.).

While groups are working on their tasks, the teacher should move from group to group, answering questions and dealing with any problems that arise. At the conclusion of the group process, some closure should take place.

Debates

Students can debate the pros and cons of many issues relating to health. Suggesting that students defend an opposing point of view provides an additional learning experience.

During a debate, each side has the opportunity to present their arguments and to refute each others' arguments. After the debate, class members can choose the side with which they agree.

Factual Writing

Once students have been presented with information about a topic, a variety of writing assignments can challenge them to clarify and express their ideas and opinions. Position papers, letters to the editor, proposals and public service announcements provide a forum in which students can express their opinions, supporting them with facts, figures and reasons.

Media Analysis

Students can analyze materials from a variety of media, including printed matter, music, TV programs, movies, video games and advertisements, to identify health-related messages. Such analysis might include identifying the purpose of the piece, the target audience, underlying messages, motivations and stereotypes.

TEACHING STRATEGIES

Personal Contracts

Personal contracts, individual commitments to changing behavior, can help students make positive changes in their health-related behaviors. The wording of a personal contract may include the behavior to be changed, a plan for changing the behavior and the identification of possible problems and support systems.

However, personal contracts should be used with caution. Behavior change may be difficult, especially in the short term. Students should be encouraged to make personal contracts around goals they are likely to meet.

Research

Research requires students to seek information to complete a task. Students may be given prepared materials that they must use to complete an assignment, or they may have to locate resources and gather information on their own. As part of this strategy, students must compile and organize the information they collect.

GLOSSARY

A

abstain—To refrain from doing something by one's own choice.

abstinence—Avoiding sexual intercourse by one's own choice.

affection—Fond or tender feeling; warm liking.

aggressiveness—Hostile, demanding, arrogant, pushy, demeaning behavior.

appropriate—Suitable for a particular occasion or situation.

assertiveness—A component of communication in which individuals stand up for what they believe, want or need, without hurting or denying the rights of others.

B

body language—A form of nonverbal communication made up of facial expressions, body movement, posture, gestures, etc., that are clues to a person's thoughts and feelings.

C

comfortable—At ease in body or mind.

communication—The ability to express thoughts, feelings and reactions and to exchange information among people through a common system of symbols, signs or behaviors.

consequence—The result of an action.

contract—An agreement between 2 or more people to do something.

culture—Ideas, customs, skills and arts of a people or group.

D

decision—The result of making up one's mind; a judgment or conclusion.

E

emotions—Feelings about or reactions to certain important events or thoughts.

F

facial expression—How the features of the face respond to emotions; a nonverbal gesture or clue that can convey how a person feels or thinks about a certain topic, idea or emotion.

G

goal—An end that a person aims to reach or accomplish.

H

heterosexual—Feeling sexual attraction toward persons of the other sex.

homosexual—Feeling sexual attraction toward persons of the same sex.

I

inappropriate—Not suitable for a particular occasion or situation.

influence—The power a person or thing has to affect others; someone or something that affects others.

intimate—Most private or personal; very close.

I-statement—A way to express thoughts, feelings and needs while respecting the rights of others.

M

mental/emotional effects—The influence something has on a person's feelings of love, hate, fear or anger.

N

norms—Standards or rules for behavior.

P

peer power—Friends influencing friends to do something positive.

peer pressure—The influence of friends on behavior; can have positive or negative results.

personal support system—Individuals who provide help or encouragement.

plan—A scheme for making, doing or arranging something; a project; a program; a schedule.

pressure lines—Statements used to persuade individuals to engage in specific activities.

psychological—Having to do with the mind, both normal and abnormal states.

R

refusal techniques—Methods of declining to do something or rejecting what is offered.

risky—Having an increased likelihood of injury, damage or other negative consequences.

risky behaviors—Actions that cause an increased likelihood of injury, damage or other negative consequences.

S

safe—Free from damage, danger or injury.

secure—Free from danger; safe; not worried or troubled.

self-esteem—Measure of how much a person values himself or herself.

sexual intercourse—A type of contact involving 1 of the following: (1) insertion of a man's penis into a woman's vagina (vaginal intercourse); (2) placement of the mouth on the genitals of another person (oral intercourse); or (3) insertion of a man's penis into the anus of another person (anal intercourse).

sexually transmitted disease (STD)—Any of a number of diseases that can spread through sexual contact.

U

unsafe—Dangerous; risky.

V

values—Beliefs or qualities that are important, desirable or prized.

RESOURCES AND REFERENCES

Resources

Videos

He's No Hero: Male Responsibility.
Examines the responsibilities of males in sexual decision making. Addresses conflicting pressures to have sex and male/female control issues in relationships (18 minutes). Available from ETR Associates.

Sexual Abstinence: Making the Right Choice.
Candid, thoughtful and persuasive commentary about abstinence from teens across the country (23 minutes). Available from ETR Associates.

Values and Choices.
Comprehensive sexuality education program that covers basic values, sexual abstinence and more. Master set includes 2 hours of video. Available from ETR Associates.

Pamphlets

Abstinence ABC's.
Provides 26 positive reasons to postpone sexual involvement. Available from ETR Associates.

Abstinence and HIV.
Includes pointers on how to stick to a policy of abstinence as protection against HIV and other sexually transmitted disease as well as unplanned pregnancy. Available from ETR Associates.

Abstinence: Think About It/Abstinencia: pieñselo.
Bilingual pamphlet explains the benefits of sexual abstinence. Available from ETR Associates.

It's About Sex!
Photopamphlet promotes honest discussion about sexual pressure. Available from ETR Associates.

Not Everyone's Doin' It!.
Photopamphlet promotes talking about abstinence. Available from ETR Associates.

101 Ways to Make Love Without Doin' It.
Offers 101 imaginative alternatives to sex. Available from ETR Associates.

101 Ways to Say No to Sex.
Offers 101 variations on saying no. Available from ETR Associates.

Positively Abstinent Teaching Kit.
Kit has 3 lessons that use colorful pamphlets to help students personalize abstinence information. Available from ETR Associates.

Sex and Abstinence.
Explains why abstinence is the only way to be 100% safe from unintended pregnancy, STD and HIV. Available from ETR Associates.

Sex? Let's Wait!
Presents realistic situations that teens can identify with and understand. Available from ETR Associates.

Sexual Responsibility: Talking with Your Teen.
Pamphlet for adults offers frank, helpful advice on communicating values and concerns. Available from ETR Associates.

Worth Waiting!
Photopamphlet encourages delaying sex and enjoying each other's company in other special ways. Available from ETR Associates.

Books

Abstinence: Health Facts. N. L. Thacker and K. R. Miner. Santa Cruz, CA: ETR Associates.
Books in the *Health Facts* series provide clear, concise background information on particular health topics, with an emphasis on topics and examples that are relevant to middle and high school students.

Self-Esteem and Mental Health: Health Facts. N. J. Krantzler and K. R. Miner. Santa Cruz, CA: ETR Associates.

Sexuality: Health Facts. L. Stang and K. R. Miner. Santa Cruz, CA: ETR Associates.

RESOURCES AND REFERENCES

Organizations

American Association of Sex
    Educators, Counselors and
    Therapists
435 N. Michigan Ave., Suite 1717
Chicago, IL 60611
(312) 644-0828

American Medical Association
Department of Health Education
515 N. State St.
Chicago, IL 60610
(800) 621-8335

American School Health Association
P.O. Box 708
Kent, OH 44240
(216) 678-1601

Centers for Disease Control and
    Prevention (CDC)
Department of Adolescent and School
    Health
4770 Buford Highway NE
Atlanta, GA 30341
(404) 488-5323

National Council for Self-Esteem
California State Department of
    Education
P.O. Box 277877
Sacramento, CA 95827
(916) 455-6273

Planned Parenthood Federation of
    America
810 Seventh Ave.
New York, NY 10019
(212) 541-7800

Sex Information and Education Council
    of the United States (SIECUS)
130 West 42nd St., Suite 2500
New York, NY 10036
(212) 819-9770

RESOURCES AND REFERENCES

References

The Alan Guttmacher Institute. 1993. *Facts in brief: Teenage sexual and reproductive behavior.* New York.

Barth, R. P. 1993. *Reducing the risk: Building skills to prevent pregnancy, STD and HIV.* 2d ed. Santa Cruz, CA: ETR Associates.

Benard, B. 1992. Fostering resiliency in kids: Protective factors in the family, school and community. *Prevention Forum* 12 (3): 13.

Berryman, J., and K. Breighner. 1994. *Modeling healthy behavior.* Santa Cruz, CA: ETR Associates.

Bridge, K. L. 1991. *Sex education for the '90s: A practical teacher's guide.* Portland, ME: J. Weston Walch.

Bruess, C., and S. Laing. 1989. *Entering adulthood: Understanding reproduction, birth and contraception.* Santa Cruz, CA: ETR Associates.

Crooks, R., and K. Baur. 1990. *Our sexuality. 4th ed.* Redwood City, CA: Benjamin/Cummings.

Fetro, J. 1992. *Personal and social skills: Understanding and integrating competencies across health content.* Santa Cruz, CA: ETR Associates.

Gordon, G. 1992. Communication. *World Book Encyclopedia.* Chicago: World Book.

Hubbard, B. 1989. *Entering adulthood: Living in relationships.* Santa Cruz, CA: ETR Associates.

Hyde, J. 1990. *Understanding human sexuality.* New York: McGraw-Hill.

Katchadourian, H. 1989. *Fundamentals of human sexuality.* 5th ed. Fort Worth, TX: Holt, Rinehart and Winston.

Krantzler, N. J., and K. R. Miner. 1994. *Self-esteem and mental health: Health facts.* Santa Cruz, CA: ETR Associates.

League of Women Voters. 1988. Attitudes toward sexuality and pregnancy. *Family Life Educator* 7 (2): 9-15.

Louis Harris and Associates. 1986. *American teens speak: Sex, myths, TV and birth control.* New York: Planned Parenthood Federation of America.

Payne, W., and D. Hahn. 1992. *Understanding your health.* 3d ed. St. Louis, MO: Mosby-Year Book.

Stang, L., and K. R. Miner. 1994. *Sexuality: Health facts.* Santa Cruz, CA: ETR Associates.

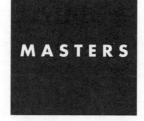

MASTERS

CONTENTS

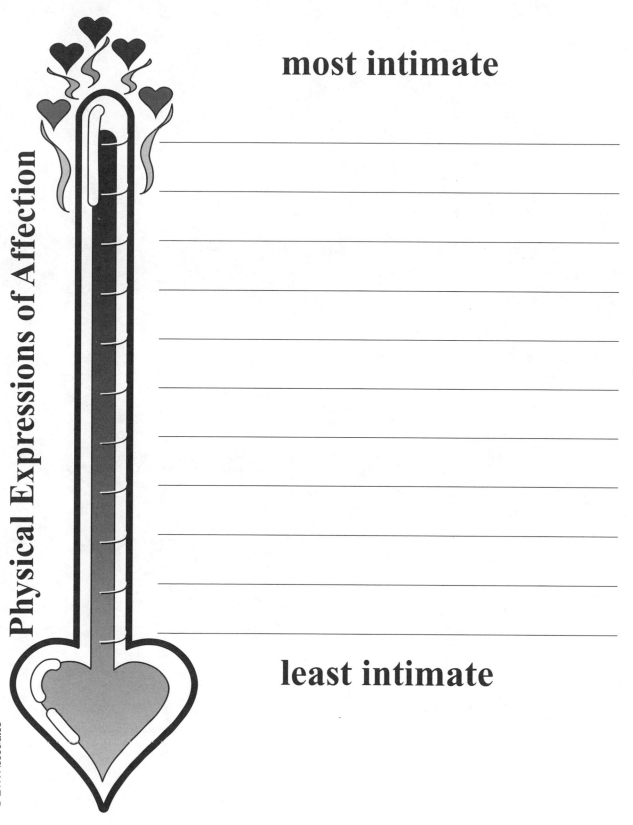

most intimate

least intimate

Physical Expressions of Affection

APPROPRIATE OR INAPPROPRIATE BEHAVIOR

Name _____ Date _____ Period _____

DIRECTIONS ➤ Read each item. Circle the **A** if the behavior is an appropriate way to express affection toward a special friend. Circle the **I** if it is inappropriate.

1. Ask someone to dance at the school dance.   **A**   **I**

2. Hold hands at a party.   **A**   **I**

3. Kiss in the school hallway.   **A**   **I**

4. Knock a person's books on the floor.   **A**   **I**

5. Write a message of love on the wall of a person's house. **A**   **I**

6. Confide a secret fear.   **A**   **I**

7. Put your arm around a person.   **A**   **I**

8. Introduce someone to your family.   **A**   **I**

9. Be alone together without adult supervision.   **A**   **I**

10. Talk about sex.   **A**   **I**

APPROPRIATE? ♥

Comprehensive Health for the Middle Grades

☐ Self-Check
☐ I read and followed directions.
☐ My work is neat and complete.
☐ This is my best work.

SELF-CHECK

TALKING ABOUT APPROPRIATE BEHAVIOR

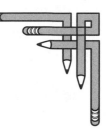

Name _____ Date _____ Period _____

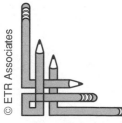

Dear Family:

Students are beginning a study of abstinence. This study is based on the philosophy that children at this age should not engage in sexual intercourse.

Today in class, students completed an activity sheet on **Appropriate and Inappropriate Behavior.** Your child has brought this activity sheet home to share with you. You may want to discuss the situations with your child. What behaviors do you think are appropriate and inappropriate for expressing affection?

You are your child's most important educator. I encourage you to share your thoughts and feelings with your child. When you disagree on subjects, try to listen to each other's perspective. If you have any questions, please call.

Sincerely,

_____

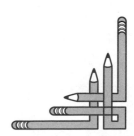

Comprehensive Health for the Middle Grades

AFFECTIONATELY YOURS

Name _____ Date _____ Period _____

DIRECTIONS ▶ For each item, write your response in the space provided.

List 5 ways you like to demonstrate your affection for a special friend.
(Examples: hug, write a nice note)

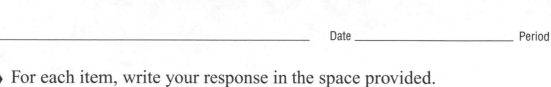

1. _____

2. _____

3. _____

4. _____

5. _____

List 5 ways students your age can have fun together.

1. _____

2. _____

3. _____

4. _____

5. _____

SELF-CHECK

☐ I read and followed directions.
☐ My ideas are clear and complete.
☐ My handwriting is readable.

Comprehensive Health for the Middle Grades

CRYSTAL BALL

Name _____ Date _____ Period _____

DIRECTIONS ▶ Under the column marked Plans, list 5 things you hope to accomplish or do in the next 6 months. Then rank your plans in order of importance from 1 (most important) to 5 (least important).

Circle any plans that would be affected if you were going to have a baby. Under the column marked Effects, explain how having a baby would affect the plans you circled.

PLANS	EFFECTS
Example: Save money for a mountain bike.	The money will go to baby needs, not the mountain bike.

☐ I read and followed directions.
☐ My ideas are clear and complete.
☐ I was honest with myself.

SELF-CHECK

SAY "WAIT" TO SEX

Name _____ Date _____ Period _____

DIRECTIONS List any reasons to avoid sexual activity from the class list that are relevant to you. Add any other reasons you have that were not mentioned in class.

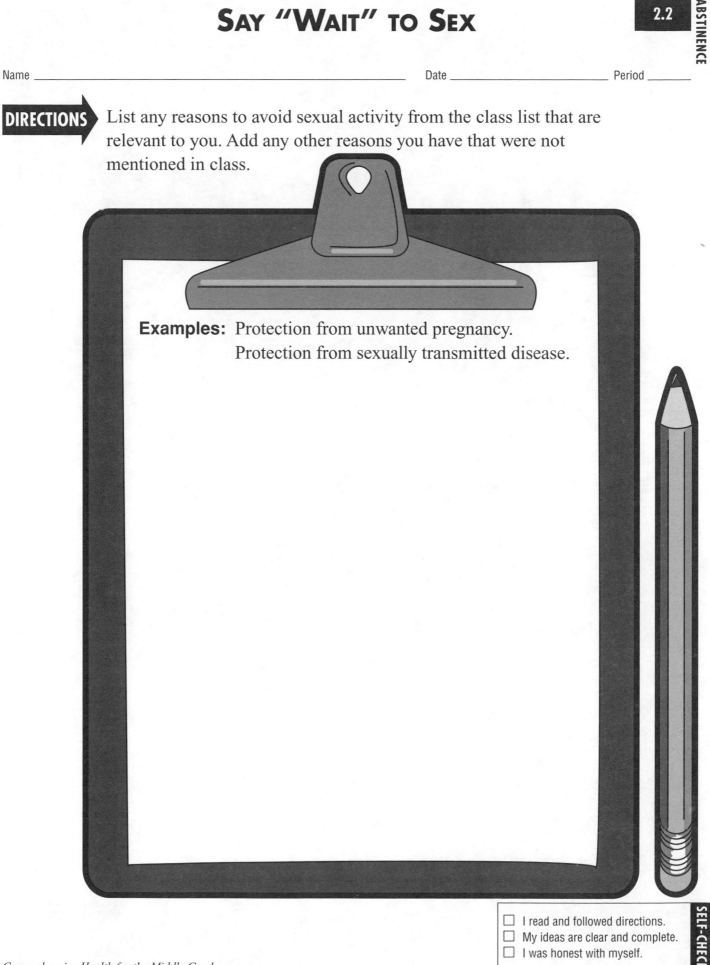

Examples: Protection from unwanted pregnancy.
Protection from sexually transmitted disease.

☐ I read and followed directions.
☐ My ideas are clear and complete.
☐ I was honest with myself.

SELF-CHECK

© ETR Associates

Comprehensive Health for the Middle Grades

REASONS TO WAIT

Name _____ Date _____ Period _____

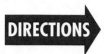 **DIRECTIONS** List the 5 best reasons why waiting until you're older to have sex is good advice for middle school students.

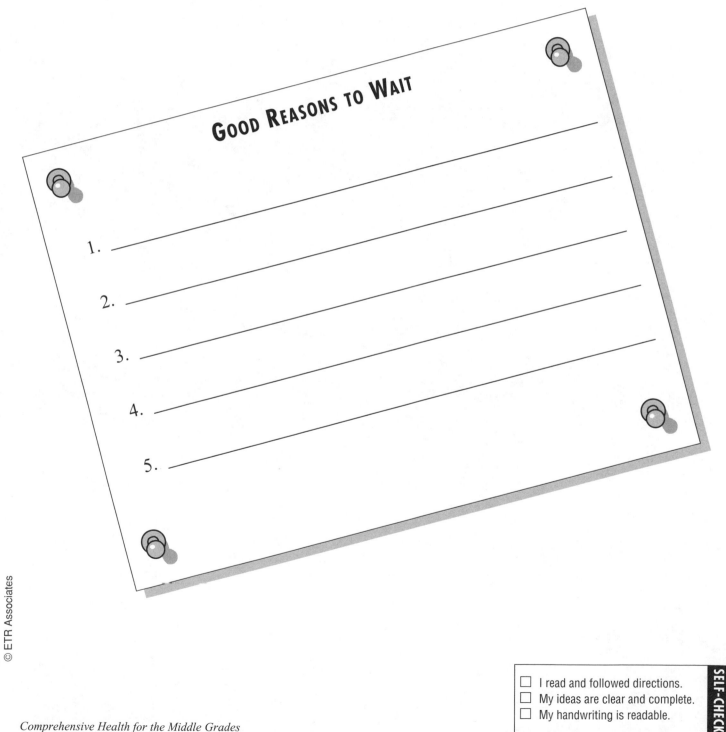

GOOD REASONS TO WAIT

1. _____

2. _____

3. _____

4. _____

5. _____

SELF-CHECK
- ☐ I read and followed directions.
- ☐ My ideas are clear and complete.
- ☐ My handwriting is readable.

CHOICES AND CONSEQUENCES

Names _____ Date _____ Period _____

DIRECTIONS Read each case study. As a group, discuss possible choices for the person. List at least 2 choices. Then discuss and list 2 possible consequences for each choice. Finally, list 1 way to have avoided the situation.

JUANITA'S CASE STUDY

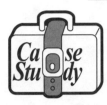

Juanita, an 8th grader, and 2 of her girlfriends went to the local high school hangout on Friday night. Juanita started talking to Carlos, a senior. Carlos invited her to go for a ride in his car. After cruising around town for a few minutes, he stopped the car and put his arm around Juanita.

What are Juanita's choices?

1. _____

_____

2. _____

_____

List 2 consequences of each choice.

1. _____

_____

_____

_____

2. _____

_____

_____

_____

How could the situation have been avoided?

_____

_____

(continued...)

CHOICES AND CONSEQUENCES

CONTINUED

JIM'S CASE STUDY

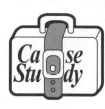

Jim, an 8th grader, was having a Halloween party. The guests, boys and girls from school, were dancing when Jim's mother and father came downstairs to see how the party was going. As soon as Jim's parents left, someone turned off the lights and the room got really dark.

What are Jim's choices?

1. _____

   _____

2. _____

   _____

List 2 consequences of each choice.

1. _____

   _____

   _____

   _____

2. _____

   _____

   _____

   _____

How could the situation have been avoided?

   _____

   _____

   _____

(continued...)

CHOICES AND CONSEQUENCES

CONTINUED

TOM'S CASE STUDY

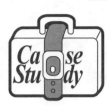

Anita, a 7th grader, invited her boyfriend Tom to her house after school to listen to a new CD. Anita lives with her father but he doesn't get home from work until 8:00 p.m. While they were listening to the music, Anita started kissing Tom.

What are Tom's choices?

1. _____

_____

2. _____

_____

List 2 consequences of each choice.

1. _____

_____

_____

_____

2. _____

_____

_____

_____

How could the situation have been avoided?

_____

_____

_____

☐ We did our best work.
☐ Our ideas are clear and complete.
☐ Everyone contributed to the group.

SELF-CHECK

Comprehensive Health for the Middle Grades

WHAT MY FAMILY THINKS

Name _____ Date _____ Period _____

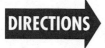**DIRECTIONS** Write your answer to the first 2 questions in class. Then take this sheet home and ask an adult family member questions 3 and 4. Write those answers in the space provided.

ASK YOURSELF

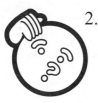
1. What are some safe settings and situations for a person my age to be in with a friend for whom I have romantic feelings?

2. What would an adult family member say are some safe settings and situations for a person my age to be in with a friend for whom I have romantic feelings?

ASK AN ADULT

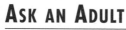
3. What are some safe settings and situations for a person my age to be in with a friend for whom I have romantic feelings?

4. When you were my age, what were considered safe settings and situations to be in with a friend for whom you had romantic feelings?

Comprehensive Health for the Middle Grades

☐ I read and followed directions.
☐ My ideas are clear and complete.
☐ My handwriting is readable.

SELF-CHECK

SHARING OPINIONS

Name _____ Date _____ Period _____

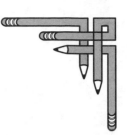

Dear Family,

An important part of abstinence is learning to avoid situations that might be conducive to sexual behavior. Examples include:

- being left alone with a special friend with no adults at home
- lying on the couch together to watch TV

Students have an activity sheet, **What My Family Thinks**, to help them identify settings and activities that support abstinence. In class, your child suggested settings he or she thought were safe and predicted what you might say.

The activity sheet has space for your responses. Please discuss with your child the kinds of situations that you consider safe for him or her. If you have any questions, please call.

Sincerely,

_____

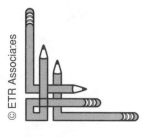

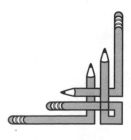

© ETR Associates

means:

✸ **expressing your feelings, needs, opinions and legitimate rights without punishing or threatening others.**

✸ **respecting yourself and others.**

PERSONAL ASSERTIVENESS INVENTORY

Name _____ Date _____ Period _____

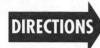 **DIRECTIONS** Read each question. Circle the letter **A**, **S** or **N** to indicate how you usually act in each situation.

A = Always act this way   S = Sometimes act this way   N = Never act this way

A S N	1. Do you keep quiet when you disagree with a friend rather than risk an argument?
A S N	2. Are you able to ask friends for help when you're confused or hurting?
A S N	3. Are you able to express your own ideas about drugs, including alcohol, even if these ideas are unpopular with your friends?
A S N	4. Do you let your friends know when they disappoint you?
A S N	5. If a friend has borrowed money and is late in paying you back, do you remind your friend?
A S N	6. Are you able to say no to a classmate who wants to copy a homework assignment that took you 2 hours to complete?
A S N	7. If you are bothered by a friend's talking and making noise during a movie, do you say so?
A S N	8. Are you able to tell a friend who always arrives 30 minutes late that you are angry?
A S N	9. Are you able to ask a friend to do a favor?
A S N	10. Are you able to refuse unreasonable requests made by a friend?
A S N	11. When you disagree with a friend, do you express your viewpoint?
A S N	12. Can you avoid doing things with your friends that you don't really want to do?

TOTAL

A ____ **S** ____ **N** ____

☐ I read and followed directions.	
☐ My work is neat and complete.	SELF-CHECK
☐ I was honest with myself.	

Comprehensive Health for the Middle Grades

Assertiveness Checklist

Name _____ Date _____ Period _____

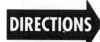 **DIRECTIONS** Fill in the roleplay name and the names of Student A and Student B for each roleplay you observe. Circle either Yes or No to answer each question. Then sign your name.

 NAME OF ROLEPLAY: _____

Name of Student A: _____
Name of Student B: _____
Did Student A…

✓ Use I-statements?	Yes	No
✓ Insist that Student B hear him or her out?	Yes	No
✓ Use a firm voice?	Yes	No
✓ Use confident body language?	Yes	No

Observer's Signature: _____

NAME OF ROLEPLAY: _____

Name of Student A: _____
Name of Student B: _____
Did Student A…

✓ Use I-statements?	Yes	No
✓ Insist that Student B hear him or her out?	Yes	No
✓ Use a firm voice?	Yes	No
✓ Use confident body language?	Yes	No

Observer's Signature: _____

NAME OF ROLEPLAY: _____

Name of Student A: _____
Name of Student B: _____
Did Student A…

✓ Use I-statements?	Yes	No
✓ Insist that Student B hear him or her out?	Yes	No
✓ Use a firm voice?	Yes	No
✓ Use confident body language?	Yes	No

Observer's Signature: _____

(continued…)

Comprehensive Health for the Middle Grades

NAME OF ROLEPLAY: _____

Name of Student A: _____

Name of Student B: _____

Did Student A…

   ✓ Use I-statements?   Yes   No

   ✓ Insist that Student B hear him or her out?   Yes   No

   ✓ Use a firm voice?   Yes   No

   ✓ Use confident body language?   Yes   No

Observer's Signature: _____

NAME OF ROLEPLAY: _____

Name of Student A: _____

Name of Student B: _____

Did Student A…

   ✓ Use I-statements?   Yes   No

   ✓ Insist that Student B hear him or her out?   Yes   No

   ✓ Use a firm voice?   Yes   No

   ✓ Use confident body language?   Yes   No

Observer's Signature: _____

NAME OF ROLEPLAY: _____

Name of Student A: _____

Name of Student B: _____

Did Student A…

   ✓ Use I-statements?   Yes   No

   ✓ Insist that Student B hear him or her out?   Yes   No

   ✓ Use a firm voice?   Yes   No

   ✓ Use confident body language?   Yes   No

Observer's Signature: _____

☐ I read and followed directions.
☐ My work is neat and complete.
☐ My handwriting is readable.

SELF-CHECK

ASSERTIVENESS PRACTICE

Name _____ Date _____ Period _____

DIRECTIONS Roleplay these situations with your group.

1. MATH HOMEWORK

Student B wants to copy Student A's math homework. Student A spent 2 hours doing this assignment.

2. AT THE MOVIES

Student A is at the movies with 3 friends. One of the friends, Student B, is talking loudly with a group of boys seated 2 rows behind. Student A can barely hear the dialogue in the movie.

3. GOING SWIMMING

Student A and Student B agree to meet Saturday morning at 9:00 to catch the bus headed downtown. Student A arrives on time at the bus stop and waits 30 minutes before Student B arrives. This is the second Saturday in a row Student B has arrived late.

4. CAN YOU COME OVER?

Last night Student A invited a good friend, Student B, to come over. Student B said he or she was sick and needed to stay home and rest. This morning at school Student A learned that Student B was at a dance last night.

SELF-CHECK
- ☐ We did our best work.
- ☐ Our ideas are clear and complete.
- ☐ Everyone contributed to the group.

Comprehensive Health for the Middle Grades

ASSERTIVENESS LOG

Name _____ Date _____ Period _____

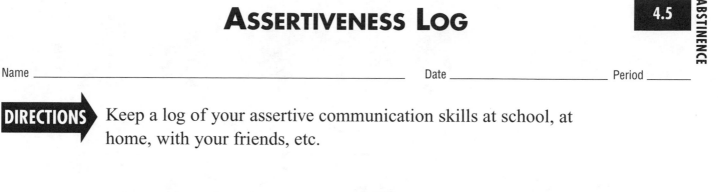

DIRECTIONS ➤ Keep a log of your assertive communication skills at school, at home, with your friends, etc.

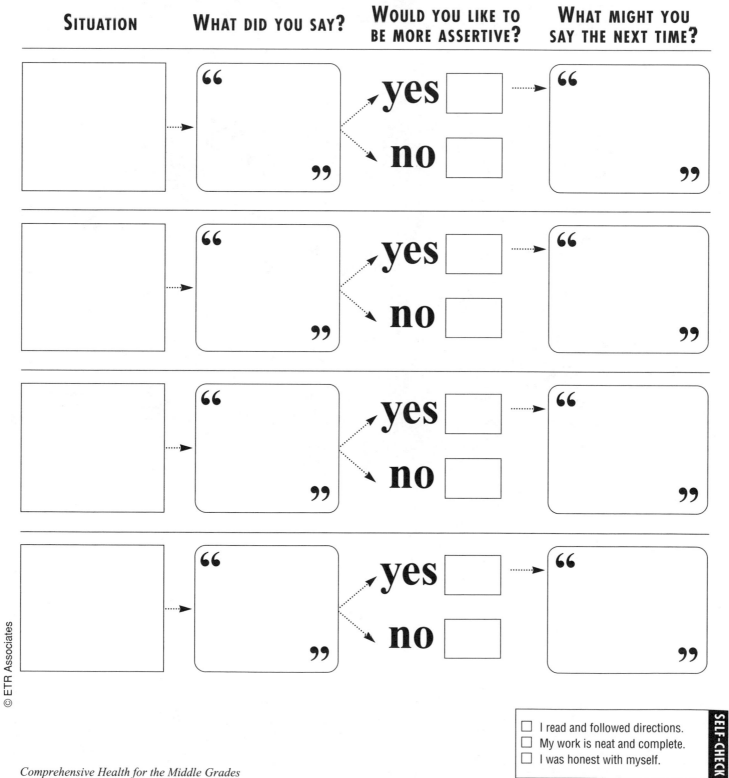

SITUATION	WHAT DID YOU SAY?	WOULD YOU LIKE TO BE MORE ASSERTIVE?	WHAT MIGHT YOU SAY THE NEXT TIME?
	" "	yes ☐ no ☐	" "
	" "	yes ☐ no ☐	" "
	" "	yes ☐ no ☐	" "
	" "	yes ☐ no ☐	" "

SELF-CHECK
☐ I read and followed directions.
☐ My work is neat and complete.
☐ I was honest with myself.

Comprehensive Health for the Middle Grades

🚫 **Say no and mean it.**

- Clearly say the word no.
- Use a firm voice.
- Use body language that says no.
- Refuse to discuss the matter any further.

🚫 **Keep saying no.**

🚫 **Give a reason.**

🚫 **Make an excuse.**

🚫 **Leave the situation.**

🚫 **Suggest something else to do.**

🚫 **Ignore the problem.**

🚫 **Make a joke of it.**

SAYING NO CHECKLIST

Name _____ Date _____ Period _____

 DIRECTIONS Fill in the pressure line and the names of Student A and Student B for each roleplay you observe. Circle either Yes or No to answer each question. Then sign your name.

PRESSURE LINE: _____

Name of Student A: _____

Name of Student B: _____

Did Student A…

✓ Clearly say the word "no"?	Yes	No		✓ Ignore the problem?	Yes	No
✓ Use a firm voice?	Yes	No		✓ Use humor?	Yes	No
✓ Repeat the word "no"?	Yes	No		✓ Use body language that said no?	Yes	No
✓ Give a reason?	Yes	No				
✓ Suggest something else to do?	Yes	No		✓ Refuse to discuss the matter any further?	Yes	No
✓ Leave the situation?	Yes	No				

CONCLUSION

Did Student A use at least 5 refusal techniques?   Yes   No

Observer's Signature: _____

PRESSURE LINE: _____

Name of Student A: _____

Name of Student B: _____

Did Student A…

✓ Clearly say the word "no"?	Yes	No		✓ Ignore the problem?	Yes	No
✓ Use a firm voice?	Yes	No		✓ Use humor?	Yes	No
✓ Repeat the word "no"?	Yes	No		✓ Use body language that said no?	Yes	No
✓ Give a reason?	Yes	No				
✓ Suggest something else to do?	Yes	No		✓ Refuse to discuss the matter any further?	Yes	No
✓ Leave the situation?	Yes	No				

CONCLUSION

Did Student A use at least 5 refusal techniques?   Yes   No

Observer's Signature: _____

(continued…)

Comprehensive Health for the Middle Grades

CONTINUED

PRESSURE LINE: _____

Name of Student A: _____

Name of Student B: _____

Did Student A…

✓ Clearly say the word "no"?	Yes	No
✓ Use a firm voice?	Yes	No
✓ Repeat the word "no"?	Yes	No
✓ Give a reason?	Yes	No
✓ Suggest something else to do?	Yes	No
✓ Leave the situation?	Yes	No

✓ Ignore the problem?	Yes	No
✓ Use humor?	Yes	No
✓ Use body language that said no?	Yes	No
✓ Refuse to discuss the matter any further?	Yes	No

CONCLUSION

Did Student A use at least 5 refusal techniques?　　　　Yes　　No

Observer's Signature: _____

PRESSURE LINE: _____

Name of Student A: _____

Name of Student B: _____

Did Student A…

✓ Clearly say the word "no"?	Yes	No
✓ Use a firm voice?	Yes	No
✓ Repeat the word "no"?	Yes	No
✓ Give a reason?	Yes	No
✓ Suggest something else to do?	Yes	No
✓ Leave the situation?	Yes	No

✓ Ignore the problem?	Yes	No
✓ Use humor?	Yes	No
✓ Use body language that said no?	Yes	No
✓ Refuse to discuss the matter any further?	Yes	No

CONCLUSION

Did Student A use at least 5 refusal techniques?　　　　Yes　　No

Observer's Signature: _____

(continued…)

PRESSURE LINE:

Name of Student A: _____

Name of Student B: _____

Did Student A…

✓ Clearly say the word "no"?	Yes	No
✓ Use a firm voice?	Yes	No
✓ Repeat the word "no"?	Yes	No
✓ Give a reason?	Yes	No
✓ Suggest something else to do?	Yes	No
✓ Leave the situation?	Yes	No

✓ Ignore the problem?	Yes	No
✓ Use humor?	Yes	No
✓ Use body language that said no?	Yes	No
✓ Refuse to discuss the matter any further?	Yes	No

CONCLUSION

Did Student A use at least 5 refusal techniques?   Yes   No

Observer's Signature: _____

PRESSURE LINE:

Name of Student A: _____

Name of Student B: _____

Did Student A…

✓ Clearly say the word "no"?	Yes	No
✓ Use a firm voice?	Yes	No
✓ Repeat the word "no"?	Yes	No
✓ Give a reason?	Yes	No
✓ Suggest something else to do?	Yes	No
✓ Leave the situation?	Yes	No

✓ Ignore the problem?	Yes	No
✓ Use humor?	Yes	No
✓ Use body language that said no?	Yes	No
✓ Refuse to discuss the matter any further?	Yes	No

CONCLUSION

Did Student A use at least 5 refusal techniques?   Yes   No

Observer's Signature: _____

SELF-CHECK

☐ We did our best work.
☐ Our ideas are clear and complete.
☐ Everyone contributed to the group.

Name _____ Date _____ Period _____

Setting the Stage

JJ and Terry have been going together for several weeks. This weekend, Terry's parents are gone. Terry's cousin is staying at the house with Terry, but has gone out to a movie. Terry is trying to convince JJ to come over.

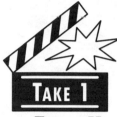

Take 1

Terry: Hey, I have a new CD. Why don't you come over so we can listen to it?

JJ: I thought your parents were out of town this weekend.

Terry: Yeah, they're gone, but my cousin is staying here. Why don't you come over now?

JJ: Is your cousin going to be there?

Terry: No, my cousin went to a movie, so we can be alone. That's OK with you, isn't it?

JJ: Well, I really would like to come over, but I don't think it's a good idea for me to be there when no one else is there.

Terry: Why not? I thought you liked me. I think it would be great to be alone.

JJ: I do like you, but I don't think it's a good idea for me to come over there now.

Terry: What's wrong with you? Nobody else would have a problem with it. You're not afraid of me, are you?

JJ: No.

Terry: Then come on over.

JJ: Well....

(continued...)

NEW CD

CONTINUED

TAKE 2

Terry: Hey, I have a new CD. Why don't you come over so we can listen to it?

JJ: I thought your parents were out of town this weekend.

Terry: Yeah, they're gone, but my cousin is staying here. Why don't you come over now?

JJ: Is your cousin going to be there?

Terry: No, my cousin went to a movie, so we can be alone. That's OK with you, isn't it?

JJ: Well, I really would like to come over, but I don't think it's a good idea for me to be there when no one else is there.

Terry: I understand. Maybe it isn't such a good idea. Why don't I bring the CD over to your house?

JJ: OK. My dad has a few friends over to watch a game on TV. We can listen to the CD in the other room.

Terry: Great, I'll be right over.

AT THE MALL

Name _____ Date _____ Period _____

DIRECTIONS ▶ Read the situation. With your group, write a dialog for this situation or for a different situation of your choice. Take 1 should show what happens if a friend doesn't respect a "no" response. Take 2 should show respect for the "no" response.

SETTING THE STAGE

You are at the mall with your boyfriend or girlfriend. You have been seeing each other for about a month. So far you have held hands and kissed. He or she says, "No one is home right now at my house. Lets go over there and turn on some music. It would give us a chance to be alone."

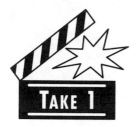

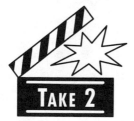

© ETR Associates

☐ We did our best work.
☐ Our ideas are clear and complete.
☐ Everyone contributed to the group.

SELF-CHECK

Comprehensive Health for the Middle Grades

Name _____ Date _____ Period _____

DIRECTIONS → Write the names and relationships to you of people who can help you abstain from sexual activity. You can list the same person more than once.

For Gathering Information About Sex

Name   *Relationship to me*

1. _____

2. _____

3. _____

For Talking About Sex

Name   *Relationship to me*

1. _____

2. _____

3. _____

SELF-CHECK
☐ I read and followed directions.
☐ My handwriting is readable.
☐ I was honest with myself.

Comprehensive Health for the Middle Grades

PEER POWER CONTRACT

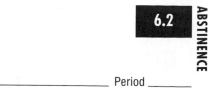

Name _____ Date _____ Period _____

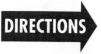 Ask a friend to support your decision to abstain from sex. Fill in and sign the contract.

DIRECTIONS Ask a friend to support your decision to abstain from sex. Fill in and sign the contract.

Date: _____

My friend, _____,
(Friend's name)
promises to help support me in my
choice to abstain from sexual activity.

_____
(Friend's signature)

_____
(My signature)

Comprehensive Health for the Middle Grades

SELF-CHECK
☐ I read and followed directions.
☐ My work is neat and complete.
☐ I was honest with myself.